The Social Construction of SARS

Discourse Approaches to Politics, Society and Culture (DAPSAC)

The editors invite contributions that investigate political, social and cultural processes from a linguistic/discourse-analytic point of view. The aim is to publish monographs and edited volumes which combine language-based approaches with disciplines concerned essentially with human interaction – disciplines such as political science, international relations, social psychology, social anthropology, sociology, economics, and gender studies.

General Editors

Ruth Wodak and Greg Myers
University of Lancaster

Editorial address: Ruth Wodak, Bowland College, Department of Linguistics and English Language, University of Lancaster University, LANCASTER LA1 4YT, UK
r.wodak@lancaster.ac.uk and g.myers@lancaster.ac.uk

Advisory Board

Volume 30

The Social Construction of SARS. Studies of a health communication crisis
Edited by John H. Powers and Xiaosui Xiao

The Social Construction of SARS

Studies of a health communication crisis

Edited by

John H. Powers
Xiaosui Xiao
Hong Kong Baptist University

John Benjamins Publishing Company
Amsterdam / Philadelphia

™ The paper used in this publication meets the minimum requirements of
American National Standard for Information Sciences – Permanence of
Paper for Printed Library Materials, ANSI z39.48-1984.

Library of Congress Cataloging-in-Publication Data

The social construction of SARS : studies of a health communication crisis / edited by
John H. Powers and Xiaosui Xiao.
    p. cm. (Discourse Approaches to Politics, Society and Culture, ISSN 1569-9463 ;
    v. 30)
  Includes bibliographical references and index.
    1. SARS (Disease) 2. Communication in public health. I. Powers, John H. (John
    Henry), 1947- II. Xiao, Xiaosui. III. Series.
    [DNLM: 1. Severe Acute Respiratory Syndrome. 2. Communication. 3. Disease
    Outbreaks. 4. Mass Media. WC 505 S6785 2008]
    RA644.S17S73   2008
362.196'2--dc22   2008030296
ISBN 978 90 272 0618 3 (Hb; alk. paper)

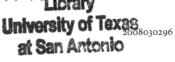

John Benjamins Publishing Co. · P.O. Box 36224 · 1020 ME Amsterdam · The Netherlands
John Benjamins North America · P.O. Box 27519 · Philadelphia PA 19118-0519 · USA

Table of contents

Introduction

John H. Powers

Hong Kong Baptist University

When the SARS virus[1] began its worldwide spread out of southern China in spring 2003, it caught regional and international health officials by surprise. Its origins were unknown, its manner of transmission was yet to be discovered, and its rapid spread was unprecedented in recent decades. First China, then Hong Kong, then several countries in East and Southeast Asia, and finally North America were all affected in rapid succession. This was truly the first international health-related crisis of the 21st century (Abraham 2004; Greenfield 2006) and, therefore, the first international health *communication* crisis as well (Ratzan 2003).

Although much has been written about the SARS crisis from economic, medical, and public health perspectives (Griffen 2005; McCright & Clark 2006; World Health Organzation 2006), relatively less has appeared from a communication perspective, though the literature is growing (see, Arquin et al. 2004; Eichelberger 2007; Ma 2005, among others identified below, for examples). However, for researchers in the health communication field, the outbreak of Severe Acute Respiratory Syndrome (SARS) provides a classic opportunity to study a large range of communication phenomena – both positive and negative – related to an unfolding public health crisis. Health care professionals, academics, government officials, news organizations, community action groups, and individual citizens around the world were all drawn into the situation, and all of them played important roles in sending, receiving, and responding to the messages aimed toward them from every direction about the emerging SARS crisis.

---

1. SARS was a particularly contagious and virulent member of the corona family of viruses that includes the virus which causes the common cold. It first appeared in humans in late 2002 in southern China. Most of the chapters in the book give additional details about the disease and its spread as they are relevant to the topic of the chapter. Other readily accessible sources about the biological and epidemiological aspects of the corona virus and SARS as a disease include Lee (2006), Sleigh (2006), and Starling (2006).

The SARS epidemic itself lasted for only few months, concluding by July 2003. However, its handling from a communication viewpoint provides important lessons that can better prepare us all for the much larger pandemic that many in the health community are predicting will occur in the not-too-distant future. In fact, as this introduction was first being prepared there were strong rumblings, first across the Asian Pacific region, and then in widely scattered locations around Europe, of a return of the H5N1 bird flu that had sporadically devastated Asian poultry industries since early 1997 and continues to kill a number of people annually who have handled infected poultry (Zhuang 2008). Avian flu was on the move via migratory birds. Moreover, there were ambiguous but worrisome signs that H5N1 might have begun to infect people via direct human-to-human transmission. Antiflu medicines were suddenly in short supply and manufacturers began making serious contingency plans for how to produce more if avian flu eventually became "the big one." Accordingly, whatever lessons there are to be learned from the SARS epidemic may need to be put to good use in the near future (for a somewhat contrarian view, see Siegel 2005).

Among the most important lessons is one that we all know at some level, but which seems to need to be relearned whenever novel circumstances like SARS confront us, namely, that the way people communicate about a topic largely determines how they are likely to understand the topic and behave toward it. In fact, a key theme in the communication literature since at least the publication of Berger and Luckman's (1966) *Social Construction of Reality* is that the specific ways of talking about something help people to construct a socially shared understanding of what they are dealing with and how best to approach it. We communicate ourselves into a particular way of thinking and acting. For example, a number of critical studies of health communication clearly show that how public discussions of specific illnesses are framed affect people's attitudes and behaviors toward those illnesses (e.g., Carter & Watney 1989; Chen & Wu 2007; Davis & Siu 2007; Elwood 1999; Fuller 2003; Fuller & Shilling 1994). Media coverage of syphilis, heart disease, lung cancer and AIDS, for instance, tend to associate the diseases with what are perceived as unhealthy lifestyles and socially disapproved conduct such as prostitution, homosexuality, and smoking. However, studies by Clarke (1992), Poirier (1995), Kisternberg (2003), among others, indicate that alternative framings of these same illnesses would have proposed different understandings and, consequently, encouraged different personal and public responses to them.

SARS was no exception. For example, in mainland China, the media largely associated the SARS outbreak with the killing of wild animals such as the paguma larvata and pangolin (e.g., *Rangwomen* 2003, May 9; *Feidian* 2003, May 20; *Hongyang* 2003, May 23; *Bushi* 2003, May 26), a pracice that still continues (Tam 2008). The media emphasized that early SARS patients had all been working closely with wild animals, either as cooks in restaurants that served game or as wild animal dealers for such restaurants. SARS was thus constructed in relation to a wild-animal-eating habit that many urban Chinese have come to think of as unhealthy and destructive to their natural environment. Following from this construction of the early cases of SARS, it seemed that nature was simply taking its rightful vengeance on human beings. Justice was being done and others need not be unduly concerned.

But, of course, they did need to be concerned. For, between November 2002 and January 2003 the SARS virus spread rapidly around southern China's Guangdong Province, then to other regions of the mainland. By February it had crossed the border into Hong Kong, and from there it spread rapidly around the world via a different kind of migratory bird, the commercial jetliner. A small moment during which an illness was constructed as being entirely local and as a proper punishment for those who were infected meant that people let their guard down at the very time a mysterious new illness was emerging among them. The fact that the communicative construction of a local illness in a far off region of China could make such a large difference in world health conditions is one of the real lessons of the SARS epidemic.

Focus and theme of the book

This book is unique in the literature on the SARS epidemic in that it brings together in one place a set of studies focused specifically on how different groups and communities socially constructed their approaches to the SARS crisis so that we can more clearly see what worked from a communication perspective and what did not. By "social construction" we specifically mean the ways people came to make sense of SARS through the ways they communicated about it. As an international epidemic, SARS arrived in a number of distinctive societies, with the result that different social constructions were fostered within those differing social and political systems, and those constructions yielded different consequences for the communities involved. Accordingly, the 12 chapters in *The Social Construction of SARS* are studies of how a major health related crisis was understood from a communication viewpoint in such diverse places as Hong Kong, mainland China, Singapore, Taiwan, Canada, and the United States during the SARS outbreak.

The central theme of the chapters is that each of the communities affected by SARS came to grips with the mysterious illness by constructing and communicating their own distinctive approaches to the crisis they were facing. Part of what the chapters reveal, when taken collectively, is that some communities were more successful than others in communicating a socially useful approach to

SARS among their citizens/audiences. Some, like Hong Kong, seem to have been relatively unsuccessful, while others such as Singapore fared much better in their health communication efforts, for reasons that our authors help to clarify.

Survey of the chapters

Most of the chapters in the book are case studies of the discursive communication practices that occurred in the communities involved. We have grouped the chapters into four Parts reflecting the country or region they most centrally feature: Hong Kong, the Chinese mainland, Singapore and Taiwan, and cross-national comparisons.

We begin with four chapters about Hong Kong, not because that is where the social construction of SARS began, but because had SARS not crossed the border into Hong Kong in February 2003, it might never have been heard about at all. Moreover, Hong Kong seems to have been the least successful in developing a satisfactory approach to its SARS-related communication, and in many ways continues to suffer from its communicative failures (Abraham 2008). Moving on from the experience of Hong Kong, the three chapters of Part II consider social constructions that arose in mainland China after the SARS genie was already out of the bottle; for, after a very unfortunate beginning to their SARS communication, Mainland officials changed their approaches and found more successful communication strategies. The three chapters of Part III feature studies of the communicative response to SARS in Singapore and Taiwan, where our authors highlight just how differently SARS communication was handled in these communities. The two chapters of the final Part are more globally comparative rather than about individual societies, with one comparing news coverage of SARS in different international regions and the other reporting on an experiment to try to determine the factors that might lead communities with different experience of SARS to interpret new information in different ways.

The purpose of the next several paragraphs is to introduce the individual chapters that make up the book and to indicate some of the connections that we find among them. For, a major lesson to be derived from the individual chapters when they are put into relationship with one another is that the way societies communicated about the unfolding health crisis made significant differences in how those communities responded, as well as to whether or not they were successful in their immediate and long-term efforts. Our ways of talking – our discursive choices – matter.

In Chapter 1, Powers and Gong consider Hong Kong's multiple constructions of SARS, analyzing five different interpretive frames about SARS that circulated in southern China and Hong Kong as the epidemic arose and developed. These five frames treated SARS, respectively, as (a) a state secret of the Chinese provincial officials, (b) a scientific mystery to be solved by the scientific community, (c) a medical epidemic that legitimized the use of emergency powers and necessitated the taking of large scale collective actions, (d) a general warning to the community concerning the poor state of Hong Kong public hygiene and, finally, as (e) a government failure that served as a catalyst for social unrest and change. For each of the frames identified, the authors indicate some of the consequences for action implied by the constructions, especially emphasizing how various constructions may compete with one another in encouraging or discouraging certain kinds of behavioral outcomes. Here, then, the emphasis in on the categories that different groups used to organize their understanding of SARS and why those verbal classifications mattered during the epidemic and beyond.

Whereas the opening chapter surveys the category-labeling terms (e.g., "state secret," "scientific mystery," and so forth) that helped frame competing interpretations of SARS, thereby providing them with a verbal center around which to coalesce, Chapter 2 reports on the storytelling done by Hong Kong's public health officials. Raising a critical question in Hong Kong's crisis communication, Xiao asks *how should a government perform its role as a public storyteller in times of grave disaster*? As Xiao argues, the Hong Kong government, which tried to communicate its response to the SARS crisis using a strictly scientific narrative about of its actions, failed to satisfy the public's need for heroic stories. Instead, the Hong Kong government's often cool and "prudent" version of scientific reporting tended to overlook the public's desire for stories celebrating great deeds done on their behalf, leaving in its wake a considerable amount of residual anger in the community long after SARS was over (Fong 2008). He argues that there is a need for heroic narratives in crisis communication to boost people's morale and reconfirm the meaning of their lives in spite of their troubles. As we will see when we describe the chapters about Singapore's communication, heroic stories were in fact presented in that community, and the outcomes in terms of social morale and support for the government's actions were much more positive (see Chapter 8 especially). Similarly, as China changed its approach from a climate of secrecy to greater openness in reporting about SARS, it too began telling stories of local heroism in the struggle against SARS, and these have contributed to a positive image of China's new generation of leaders (see Chapter 6 in particular). So, it would appear that citizens do indeed respond to the kinds of storytelling that their leaders choose to perform.

There are many dimensions or levels of language that contribute to the construction of a phenomenon as complex as SARS. As we saw above, one of those dimensions includes the verbal frames people use to organize their intepretations of an event, and another is the stories that are told about the actions of those in power. In Chapter 3, Gong and Dragga focus special attention on a different dimension, namely, the lexical level of language, by examining the political and economic concerns that appear to have influenced Hong Kong's public health officials to use interchangeably two different labels for the new disease: *SARS* and *atypical pneumonia*. Regrettably, the acronym used by the World Health Organization (WHO) for the epidemic, *SARS*, happened to overlap with the official acronym for Hong Kong as a Special Administrative Region (SAR) of China. The Hong Kong government perceived the uniform application of the SARS acronym, a globally recognized name, as politically embarrassing. Gong and Dragga's study reveals that public health officials tended to use the categorical labeling term *atypical pneumonia* long after it was medically accurate to do so. However, the use of that politically safe term proved to be medically unsafe because it resulted in a serious delay of the implementation of quarantine measures that might have reduced the early spread of the disease. Thus, the lesson learned from Gong and Dragga's chapter is that something so small as the way a new disease is named can have consequences for the community involved, especially when that name has the potential for creating politically sensitive issues.

Where people get their news makes a difference because of the various pressures on different news sources and what they are permitted to report. Chapter 4 explores the role of news Web sites in Hong Kong and mainland China during the SARS crisis. In this comparative study, Lee indicates that news sites originating in Hong Kong, which enjoy a high degree of Internet press freedom, acted as "interactive crisis managers" and contributed in a number of ways to reporting and managing the crisis in the community. In contrast, news sites in mainland China, which were restricted by media censorship, served as the government's "online agent of containment." What Lee's study suggests, then, is that press freedom contributes to wider access to alternate constructions and therefore promotes greater freedom of choice in how one responds to a crisis such as SARS. Thus, it is not just that press freedom can provide more information, but also that it can enable different ways of understanding the information that is actually available.

The chapters of Part II move from studies of Hong Kong communication about SARS to those concerned with mainland China's communication. Chapter 5 presents a qualitative analysis of the SARS-related stories covered in the *People's Daily*, an organ of the Chinese Communist Party not subject to the economic pressures of the marketplace, and *Beijing Youth News*, a relatively market-oriented newspaper which is still ultimately subject to Communist Party oversight. Huang and Hao's analysis reveals that the two newspapers, despite their need to adhere to the Party's overall policy towards information management during the epidemic, differed in the presentation of their stories in a number of features, including how much time was spent quoting Party officials, the degree to which human interest stories were included in the reporting, and even differences in the possibility of covertly suggesting information that could be read between the lines. In a nation where the ability to control the flow of information limits the types of constructive understandings the people might be able to generate, the differences between the two newspapers suggests an ongoing struggle within China at many levels. For, as Huang and Hao report, the newspapers subject to commerical pressures tell their stories in substantially different ways from those that are not, even where the underlying imperative is to promote the Communist Party's essential line.

Chapter 6 takes a more rhetorical approach to the anti-SARS campaign in mainland China. Based on an examination of the "fantasy themes" of character, action, and setting that were expressed in the language of popular books about the crisis, Lu finds that through positive portrayals of national leaders and vivid depictions of the heroic acts of medical workers a renewed sense of nationalism was constructed, one characterized by patriotism and sacrifice for the Party and country. Thus, Lu argues that China's anti-SARS discourse fostered a rhetorical vision of national unity, so that the discourse promoted simultaneously both nationalism and reinvigorated traditional Chinese cultural values. In mainland China, fighting against SARS became another meaning-filled campaign of nationalism and patriotism. The anti-SARS campaign thus was socially and politically significant for the Communist Party because it not only provided the Party with a crucial opportunity to show its administrative competence but also to re-establish the legitimacy of its moral governance at a time of both national crisis and a transition to a new generation of political leadership. As one might already realize, the difference between Hong Kong's approach to communicating about SARS, as described in Chapter 2, and Lu's description of Mainland popular approaches, puts the issue of the social importance of heroic portrayals during a crisis into stark relief.

When looking at the language of SARS, sometimes the devil is truly in the details. Accordingly, Chapter 7 provides a very focused critical discourse analysis of a series of daily SARS case reports that were provided by the News Office of the Health Ministry of China beginning on April 21, the day immediately after Minister Zhang Wenkang was dismissed as its director (see Zhang & Benoit, in press, for more details). Tian's analysis shows how the news reports changed from day to day, as well as over the course of a month of reporting, so that the information structure of the reports served to construct a particular anti-SARS ideology in favor of the Ministry of Health's position on SARS developments. It did this by attaching prominence to information that agreed with the interests and beliefs of the Ministry and downgrading the information that did not. The Ministry's particular anti-SARS ideology was evolved every day as information (defined by Tian in terms of "stages" of unfolding) was selectively included or excluded in the daily reports so that reporters were subtly influence to report stories that reflected well on the government's fight against SARS. For readers interested in the finer details of language analysis and how those details might influence an audience's perception of an event such as SARS, this will be a particularly useful chapter.

Chapter 8, the first of the three chapers of the book's third Part, investigates how the Singapore media worked along with the government to mobilize the nation during the SARS crisis by emphasizing Confucian ethics. Weber, Tan and Law present a discourse analysis based on articles that were published by Singapore's flagship daily newspaper the *Straits Times* during the crisis. In the authors' view, *crisis* has long been a recurrent theme of the Singapore government's nationalistic discourse. The ruling People's Action Party has historically constructed Singapore as a society and nation in crisis, as being "a vulnerable and reluctant small nation after the traumatic expulsion from the union with Malaysia in 1965." The emergence of SARS thus enabled the Singaporean government to reinforce its extant discourse of crisis and nation. Weber, Tan and Law show that the media contributed significantly to enriching Singapore's national mythology of "triumph over adversity" that ties citizens to national goals. This chapter serves as a sort of supporting evidence for the claim in Chapter 2 that Hong Kong's lack of heroic narratives harmed the government's effectiveness and reputation. For, in Singapore, such narratives were part of a relatively successful community campaign that actually helped to rebuild the government's flagging image among a sizeable portion of its citizens.

In Chapter 9 Hudson presents a critical rhetorical analysis of the Singapore government's campaign against SARS. In Hudson's view the government applied a war metaphor to introduce fear, heroes, victory, and national pride, while also using it to obscure the increased surveillance, militarization, and authoritarianism that were employed during the SARS crisis. The spread of SARS in Singapore became a public spectacle in which a deadly illness was metaphorically transmuted into a threat to the integrity of the nation. For Singaporeans, the "War on SARS" entered the popular imagination in parallel with the war in Iraq, thereby invoking the language of military strength, a community united in adversity, the defence of national borders, and the threat of a pestilence that had the potential to kill the economy. Thus, Hudson's chapter examines the ways in which SARS acquired metaphorically charged meaning beyond the basic epidemiological concerns, and it argues that successful eradication of the disease became a "defining moment" in the history of Singapore, bringing about a resurgence of national identity. The importance of metaphors in understanding diseases such as SARS, especially war metaphors that promote the "fight" against these diseases, has been highlighted in several recent publications (Baehr 2006; Chaing & Duann 2007; Nerlich & Halliday 2007; Wallis & Nerlich 2005), so that Hudson's chapter is both a welcome contribution to that general body of literature and also a thoughtful case study of the role that metaphor played in the Singapore experience of SARS in particular.

Although there is a relatively large and growing literature on the news coverage of the SARS epidemic (see, for example, Beaudoin 2007; Berry, Wharf-Higgens, & Naylor 2007; Lee 2005; Leung & Huang 2007; Meng & Berger 2008; Tai & Sun 2007; Tian & Stewart 2005; Washer 2004; Wilkins 2005; Huang & Leung 2005; Zhang & Fleming 2005), most of it looks at what the papers reported and how they reported it. None has previously examined the behind-the-scenes struggles and conflicts that SARS reporters faced as the crisis began to move so quickly that the daily deadlines put pressures on accuracy, completeness, and even human resources. Accordingly, Chapter 10 represents a major contribution to our understanding of SARS news coverage by presenting a journalist's perspective on SARS health communication reporting. Based on in-depth interviews with a number of frontline medical journalists from the mainstream Taiwanese news media, Hsu seeks to explain how SARS news was produced in Taiwan and why the stories published were so roundly criticized as inadequate, filled with misinformation, and poorly presented. For anyone who has ever criticized the news coverage of fast-moving events, this chapter will provide insights into the processes and pressures that contribute to what eventually gets put onto the printed page.

Also exploring mass mediated disease reporting, Chapter 11 by Houston, Chao and Ragan, examines how media in different societies defined and constructed SARS for their audiences in communities that had quite different experiences with SARS. The authors conducted a content analysis of newspaper articles drawn from the *New York Times*, Hong Kong's *South China Morning Post*, the *Toronto Star*, and Malaysia's *New Straits Times*, and focused their examination on the topics covered in each paper, the news sources cited, and the types of frames used in their coverage of the SARS outbreak. Among several interesting findings, the authors discover that Hong Kong's *South China Morning Post* included the most articles that criticized the public policies that were implemented to handle the crisis, whereas Malaysia's *New Straits Times* had the most articles that lauded public officials for their handling the SARS outbreak. The *Toronto Star* placed more emphasis on the economic impact of SARS, and related issues. The results also indicate a strong influence of government on media construction – given that government sources were found to be the most frequently utilized in the overall media coverage in all locations.

The book's final chapter is concerned with how personal cognitive style interacts with the attributes of a news story in the processing of risk information. Contributing to a body of social scientific literature on SARS (see, for example,

Guo, Cheong & Shen 2005), Zhou, Pan and Zhong conducted experiments respectively in the United States and China, using identical manipulations and measurement instruments, to discover how social perception and the construction of social reality are interlinked. The tests suggest that news story attributes consistently affected story evaluation. In particular, story context information played an important role in assuaging SARS apprehension for participants with a proclivity for rational processing. Based on this research the authors suggest several implications for action when health officials need to convey critical information to various constituencies within their communities; moreover, their conclusion brings us back full circle to the role that interpretive frames played in the SARS communication process and its consequences.

In sum, then, the chapters that follow not only provide a detailed analysis of the communication that occurred during a large health crisis but also point the way to many principles related to how community leaders might conduct their communication efforts as they plan their health related campaigns in the future. Certainly, getting scientific information out to the public in a timely manner is a must. But so are adequate framings of the illness, stories of the heroic efforts of those on the front line, and galvanizing metaphors that can bind the community together even when the illness is unpredictable and the chances of scientific success are uncertain. My co-editor and I hope you enjoy the volume and find many useful ideas in every chapter.

References

Abraham, T. (2004). *Twenty-first century plague: The story of SARS*. Hong Kong: Hong Kong University Press.

Abraham, T. (2008, March 25). Communication lessons from Sars go to waste. Letters to the Editor, *South China Morning Post*, p. A11.

Arquin, P. M., Navin, A. W., Steele, S. F., Weld, L. H., & Kozarsky, P. E. (2004). Health communication during SARS. *Emerging Infectious Diseases, 10*(2), 377–380.

Baehr, P. (2006). Susan Sontag, battle language and the Hong Kong SARS outbreak of 2003. *Economy and Society, 35*, 42–64.

Beaudoin, C. E. (2007). SARS news coverage and its determinants in China and the US. *International Communication Gazette, 69*, 509–524.

Berger, P. L., & Luckmann, T. (1966). *The social construction of reality: A treatise in the sociology of knowledge*. Garden City, NY: Doubleday.

Berry, T.-R., Wharf-Higgins, J., & Naylor, P. J. (2007). SARS wars: An examination of the quantity and construction of health information in the news media. *Health Communication, 21*, 35–44.

Bushi yesheng dongwu, koufu haishi kou huo (Is it luck or disaster to kill and eat wild animals?) (2003, May 27). *Fazhi Ribao* (Legality Daily). Retrieved May 27 2003, from http://libwisenews.wisers.net/wisenews/content.co?wp_dispatch=document&doc-id=news:20.

Carter, E., & Watney, S. (Eds.). (1989). *Taking liberties: AIDS and cultural politics*. London: Serpent's Tail.

Chaing, W.-Y., & Duann, R.-F. (2007). Conceptual metaphors for SARS: "War" between whom? *Discourse & Society, 18,* 579–602.

Chen, G., & Wu, C. (2007). A tale of two crises: SARS and AIDS. In S. Hom & S. Moser (Eds.), *Challenging China: Struggle and hope in an era of change.* New York: Human Rights in China.

Clarke, J. N. (1992). Cancer, heart disease, and AIDS: What do the media tell us about these diseases? *Health Communication, 4,* 105–120.

Davis, D., & Siu, H. (Eds.). (2007). *SARS: Reception and Interpretations in three Chinese cities.* New York: Routledge.

Eichelberger, L. (2007). SARS and New York's Chinatown: The politics of risk and blame during an epidemic of fear. *Social Science & Medicine, 65,* 1284–1295.

Elwood, W. (1999). *Power in the blood: A handbook on AIDS, politics, and communication.* Mahwah, NJ: Erlbaum.

Feidian yu huanjing xingwei miqiexiangguan (Atypical pneumonia is closely related to our environmental behavior) (2003, May 20). *Renmin Ribao* (People's Daily), p. 16.

Fong, L. (2008, February 25). Living in the shadows. *South China Morning Post*, p. A12.

Fuller, L. K. (Ed.). (2003). *Media-mediated AIDS.* Cresskill, NJ: Hampton Press.

Fuller, L. K., & Shilling, L. M. (1994). *Communicating about communicable diseases.* Amherst, MA: HRD Press.

Greenfield, K. T. (2006). *China syndrome: The true story of the 21st century's first great epidemic.* New York: HarperCollins.

Griffen, A. S. (Ed.). (2005). *Progress in SARS research.* New York: Nova Biomedical Books.

Guo, S. Z., Cheong, A. W. H., & Shen, F. C. (2005). Depth of reasoning and information processing: A predictive model of SARS behavior. *Asian Journal of Communication, 15,* 274–288.

Health Canada (2003). *Learning from SARS.* Retrieved October 20 2003 from http://www.hc-sc.gc.ca/english/pdf/sars/sars-e.pdf.

Hongyang shengtai wenming, baohu shengwu duoyangxing (Enrich our ecology, maintain the diversity of living beings) (2003, May 23). *Renmin Ribao* (People's Daily), p. 11.

Huang, Y., & Leung, C. M. (2005). Western-led press coverage of Mainland China and Vietnam during the SARS crisis: Reassessing the concept of "media representation of the other." *Asian Journal of Communication, 15,* 302–318.

Kisternberg, C. (2003). The voice of reason? A political construction of AIDS. In L. K. Fuller (Ed.), *Media-mediated AIDS* (pp. 11–22). Cresskill, NJ: Hampton Press.

Kleinman, A., & Watson, J. L. (Eds.). (2006). *SARS in China: Prelude to pandemic?* Stanford, CA: Stanford University Press.

Lee, A. Y. L. (2005). Between global and local: The glocalization of online news coverage on the transregional crisis of SARS. *Asian Journal of Communication, 15,* 255–273.

Lee, S. H. (Ed.). (2006). *SARS in China and Hong Kong.* New York: Novinka.

Leung, C. C. M., & Huang, Y. (2007). The paradox of journalistic representation of the other: The case of SARS coverage on China and Vietnam by western-led English-language media in five countries. *Journalism, 8,* 675–697.

Ma, R. (2005). Media, crisis, and SARS: An introduction. Special Edition, *Asian Journal of Communication, 15*, 241–246.

McCright, A. M., & Clark, T. M. (2006). The political ecology of plague in the global network of cities: The SARS epidemic of 2002–2003. In A. M. McCright & T. M. Clark (Eds.), *Community and ecology: Dynamics of place, sustainability and politics*. Amsterdam; Oxford: Elsevier JAI.

Meng, J., & Berger, B. K. (2008). Comprehensive dimensions of government intervention in crisis management: A qualitative content analysis of news coverage of the 2003 SARS epidemic in China. *China Media Research, 4*(1), 19–28.

Nerlich, B., & Halliday, C. (2007). Avian flu: The creation of expectations in the interplay between science and the media. *Sociology of Health & Illness, 29*, 46–65.

Poirier, S. (1995). *Chicago's war on syphilis, 1937–1940: The times, the Trib, and the clap doctor.* Urbana: University of Illinois Press.

Rangwomen li yesheng dongwu geng yuan yixie (Let's stay further away from wild animals) (2003, May 9). *Renmin Ribao* (People's Daily), p. 14.

Ratzan, S. C. (2003). Putting SARS in perspective: A communication challenge. *Journal of Health Communication, 8*, 297–298.

Shenzhen shi renmin daibiao dahui changwu weiyuanhui gonggao (The 90th Announcement of the People's Congress Standing Committee) (2003, September 8). Retrieved December 22, 2004, from http://www.southen.com/law/fzzt/fgsjk/200412220985.htm.

Siegel, M. (2005). *False alarm: The truth about the epidemic of fear.* Hoboken, NJ: John Wiley & Sons.

Sleigh, A. C. (Ed.). (2006). *Population dynamics and infectious diseases in Asia.* Singapore: World Scientific.

Starling, A. (Ed.). (2006). *Plague, SARS and the story of medicine in Hong Kong.* Hong Kong: Hong Kong University Press.

Tam, F. (2008, February 26). No health fears as diners seek wild game on thriving black market. *South China Morning Post*, p. A14.

Tambyah, P., & Leung, P.-C. (Eds.). (2006). *Bird flu: A rising pandemic in Asia and beyond?* Singapore: World Scientific.

Tai, Z., & Sun, T. (2007). Media dependencies in a changing media environment: The case of the 2003 SARS epidemic in China. *New Media and Society, 9*, 987–1009.

Tian, Y., & Stewart, Concetta, M. (2005). Framing the SARS crisis: A computer-assisted text analysis of CNN and BBC online news reports of SARS. *Asian Journal of Communication, 15*, 289–301.

University of Hong Kong Public Opinion Programme Web Site press release. Retrieved March 11, 2003, from http://hkupop.hku.hk/english/archive/release/release92.html.

Wallis, P., & Nerlich, B. (2005). Disease metaphors in new epidemics: The UK media framing of the 2003 SARS epidemic. *Social Science and Medicine, 60*, 2629–2639.

Washer, P. (2004). Representations of SARS in British newspapers. *Social Science & Medicine, 59*, 2561–2571.

Wilkins, L. (2005). Plagues, pestilence and pathogens: The ethical implications of news reporting of a world health crisis. *Asian Journal of Communication, 15*, 247–254.

World Health Organization. (2006). *How a global epidemic was stopped.* Geneva: World Health Organization, Western Pacific Region.

Zhang, E., & Benoit, W. L. (in press). Former Minister Zhang's Discourse on SARS: Government's Image Restoration or Destruction? In W. L. Benoit (Ed.). In Press. Cresskill, NJ: Hampton Press.

Zhang, E., & Fleming, K. (2005). Examination of characteristics of news media under censorship: A content analysis of selected Chinese newspapers' SARS coverage. *Asian Journal of Communication, 15,* 319–339.

Zhang, W. K. (2003, April 3). Press Conference on SARS by Health Minister Zhang Wenkang. Retrieved October 2, 2003, and October 9, 10, and 13, 2004, from http://www.china-un.ch/eng/46627.html.

Zhuang, P. (2008, February 22). 19th bird-flu victim on mainland. *South China Morning Post,* p. A10.

PART I

Constructions of SARS in Hong Kong

CHAPTER 1

Hong Kong's multiple constructions of SARS

John H. Powers and Gwendolyn Gong
Hong Kong Baptist University / Chinese University of Hong Kong

This chapter identifies five significant interpretive frames which operated in Hong Kong and southern China as the SARS crisis developed in spring 2003. These five frames treated SARS, respectively, as (a) a state secret of the Chinese provincial officials, (b) a scientific mystery to be solved by the scientific community, (c) a medical epidemic that legitimized the use of emergency powers and necessitated the taking of large scale collective actions, (d) a general warning to the community concerning the poor state of public hygiene and, finally, as (e) a government failure that served as a catalyst for social unrest and change. As each frame is described some of the behavioral and actional consequences of using the frame are also indicated.

Although outbreaks of SARS occurred in many places around the world, Hong Kong was not only hit early, it was also hit among the hardest in terms of the number of cases reported and the number of deaths recorded. As residents of Hong Kong ourselves, we remember waking up each morning from March through June wondering what the overnight news would bring and how we should understand what the government, the health care workers, and our fellow citizens were doing – as face masks were donned, classes were cancelled, businesses were closed (often never to reopen), and travel plans were rethought, replaced, and rerouted.

When people try to understand important phenomena such as the outbreak of SARS in Hong Kong, they typically construct an interpretive frame into which the information they receive is adapted to fit so that it can make coherent sense. An interpretive frame may be defined as an overall way of understanding a phenomenon, especially by putting it into a category one already understands and has previously developed a way to respond to (Tannen 1993). That is, we give the new phenomenon a name that tells us what we are talking about. This process is like building the outer border of a jigsaw puzzle that one puts together first and which subsequently provides a way of placing the rest of the pieces to form a coherent pattern or picture. From a communication viewpoint, interpretive frames are usually signaled by the broadest categories communicators use to talk about a phenomenon: it is a *crisis*, a *tragedy*, a *mystery*, *witchcraft*, and so forth.

Once a frame has been constructed and coded in such categorical terms, other communication phenomena, such as metaphors, propositional statements, presuppositions, speech acts, definitions, narratives, descriptions, arguments, and the like, are all adopted and adjusted to one another so that they are coherent among themselves and reflective of the overall interpretive frame within which they operate. However, the more information that is subsumed to the interpretive frame as we build it up, the more difficult it becomes to see the phenomenon from alternative viewpoints, however inadequate or harmful the interpretive frame we have built may happen to be, and however many other competing interpretive frames may also exist within the larger community. Identifying the interpretive frames that are being used by various groups to understand a phenomenon such as SARS is important because people take future-oriented action based on how they have constructed their framework for understanding the past and present. That is, once a group of people adopt a particular interpretive frame, they may be expected to choose their subsequent behaviors in terms of it. It provides them with a guide to action as well as a basis for abstract understanding.

Our experience of the SARS epidemic while living in Hong Kong has led us to consider the multiple interpretive frames that were constructed and used as the crisis developed over a period of little less than five months.

Five constructions of SARS

In this chapter, we will describe five such frames or symbolic constructions of SARS that seem to have had implications for how different major groups within the Hong Kong community responded to the crisis. These five frames treated SARS, respectively, as (a) a state secret of the Chinese provincial officials, (b) a scientific mystery to be solved by the scientific community, (c) a medical epidemic that legitimized the use of emergency powers and necessitated the taking of large scale collective actions, (d) a general warning to the community concerning the poor state of public hygiene and, finally, as (e) a government failure that served as a catalyst for social unrest and change.

SARS as a state secret of Chinese provincial officials

It is generally accepted that the outbreak of SARS began in southern China's city of Foshan in mid-November 2002, that the disease quickly radiated outward and gradually spread Northward throughout December and January, and that by the third week of January the Guangzhou Department of Health had received a confidential report about the outbreak in the southern Guangdong region, so that relevant officials clearly understood that they had a developing epidemic on their hands that they could not control. According to a chronology prepared by Chiu and Galbraith (2004), only a week later a SARS patient arrived in the provincial capital of Guangzhou where he infected as many as 56 people in two hospitals, which was in addition to 19 members of his own family he had infected previously. In spite of this, and the fact that people in Guangdong province had been wearing facemasks and fumigating their homes with boiling vinegar for weeks, the provincial authorities notified the central authorities only on February 8 and held a press conference in Guangdong on February 10 to reassure people that everything was under control. Chiu and Galbraith indicate that the outbreak was reported to the World Health Organization (WHO) the next day, but suggest that the report minimized its seriousness. It is also generally accepted that those same local officials did not directly share this information with Hong Kong authorities until after the first case had crossed the border on February 21, 2003, and began an epidemic there.

Based on these facts, we may wonder what possible interpretation of the alarming events in southern China might have led local officials to be so unwilling to share the information they had available with either the central government, the WHO, or with the parallel health officials in Hong Kong, whose health and safety were subsequently put at such terrible risk? The answer appears to be related to how Guangdong health and political officials constructed an understanding of their responsibility within the Chinese bureaucratic system. According to White (2003),

> Rulers in China for millennia held an odd belief: that natural disasters, such as earthquakes or new diseases, reflect on their legitimacy. Guangdong cadres repressed news of early cases of SARS out of fear that knowledge of this mysterious illness would disturb the populace and sow "disorder" (*luan*).   (p. 31)

If this observation is correct, Hong Kong officials were kept in the dark because to acknowledge that Guangdong province had an uncontrolled epidemic on its hands would have been to risk the loss of face of the provincial officials involved. Their fitness to rule (and, especially, their ability to keep their positions) would have been challenged because their very job description was to maintain the appearance of stability in the territory under their jurisdiction. SARS was, therefore, constructed essentially as a mandate from heaven indicating their *unfitness* for service. Moreover, the officials involved apparently failed to share the relevant information with virtually everyone who should have known, not just their nearest neighbors in Hong Kong (McNally 2003). For example, White (2003) observes:

> Evidence suggests that top Beijing politicos did not hear about SARS as a serious disease until February 2003, and that provincial cadres – notable Guangdong Party Secretary Zhang Dejiang – suppressed both public and governmental reporting until it could no longer be hidden.
>
> (p. 43)

Although much more might be said about the tendency toward state secrecy in China's response to SARS in the early days (more openness prevailed from late March onward as new leadership at the top began to assert itself),[1] the point we wish to make here is that for the Guangdong officials involved, the construction of SARS as a challenge to their political legitimacy (and therefore a danger to their bureaucratic survival) prevented them from treating the growing epidemic as a threat to the very people whose wellbeing they were responsible for protecting. The traditional political frame within which they operated blinded them from doing what would seem on the surface to be the only responsible thing to do, namely, acknowledging that an emerging situation was getting out of hand and seeking help from higher authorities. Here, then, we have an instance of where an interpretive frame motivated actions (including severe press clampdowns designed to enforce the secrecy) that were counterproductive to sharing the kind of information that might have prevented the worldwide spread of the disease and thereby reduced the eventual death toll caused.

SARS as a scientific mystery

The second interpretive frame we would like to feature concerning SARS arose in the scientific community, and it had a completely different effect on the behavior within that group than the construction of SARS as a state secret had on Chinese provincial authorities. For the scientific community, discovering the nature of the causative agent of SARS was a tremendous scientific mystery to be solved through a vigorous sharing of information among their peers within the microbiological community. It is not that scientists are never secretive about their research. After all, there are professional jealousies concerning who makes certain discoveries "first," prizes and awards to be distributed for contributing to the advancement of knowledge, academic promotions and lucrative patents to take into account as one decides what to share and when to share it; and there are, of course, public humiliations to avoid in cases where a particular line of research proves to be on the wrong track. The contest between Jonas Salk and Albert Sabin to create the

---

1.   Chapter 4 by Lee (this volume) is particularly helpful in shedding additional light on this constructive frame.

first polio vaccine in the 1950s is a classic case of the contest of professional egos battling it out in an important parallel situation.

The horserace tensions that can motivate research scientists on the cutting edge of the scientific quest to solve the mysteries of SARS is hinted at by Seno and Reyes (2003), when they write that:

> This discovery [that SARS belonged to the corona virus family], announced by HKU on 21 March, generated considerable excitement within the international scientific community and did much to showcase Hong Kong's research capacity. While labs in Canada and the US completed the genetic sequencing of the SARS virus first, Hong Kong's microbiologists were not far behind, their efforts validating other results. The SARS outbreak also highlighted the excellence of Hong Kong's healthcare system. Two teams of doctors from the SAR were the first to publish scientific reports describing SARS symptoms and indicators as well as treatments. Health professionals elsewhere closely watched how Hong Kong's healthcare workers were treating SARS patients in order to learn how to deal with their own cases.   (p. 12)

In the case of the SARS microbial mystery, however, considerations that might have led to scientific secrecy and jealousy were apparently set aside for the sake of solving the scientific mystery as rapidly as possible. According to Chan-Yeung and Loh (2003), virologist Klaus Stohr of the WHO was the motivating force in constructing an interpretive framework that invited the collective efforts of multiple laboratories around the world to cooperate on solving the SARS mystery without internecine strife.

> Stohr was the mastermind behind the network. He invited the world's top research laboratories to do something unprecedented – to collaborate in a virtual global laboratory. Scientists at the three Hong Kong institutions involved in the consortium – HKU, the Chinese University of Hong Kong (CUHK) and the Department of Health – were among the first to agree to cooperate. Stohr carefully selected which laboratories to tap, taking into account the expertise of each research team. . . .
> The priority for the virus hunters was speed. With the virus spreading quickly, Stohr needed answers fast. If he had been forced to wait for each research team to come up with its own results, it would have taken considerably longer than if the teams worked together. "We needed people to share data and set aside Nobel Prize interests or their desire to publish articles," Stohr said.   (p. 46)

What Chan-Yeung and Loh's remarks highlight is the behavioral consequences of treating SARS as a public scientific mystery to be solved rather than a dirty little secret to be hidden from both the public whom it affects and the higher level officials who have the power to authorize the resources needed to tackle the problems involved. By treating the unknown dimensions of the SARS virus as a scientific mystery to be unraveled rather than as an embarrassing and delegitimizing failure of scientific leadership or insight, the scientific community was able to quickly mobilize widely scattered laboratory resources and various types of virological expertise around a commonly shared intellectual and practical challenge. By framing SARS as an immediately relevant and pressingly urgent scientific mystery, the scientific community was able to overcome any tendency it may have had toward its own distinctive forms of secrecy in the name of "being first" in order to synthesize the globally distributed expertise into a "superlab" that created a very unusual and synergistic team of researchers in spite of the global distances involved. The ultimate result of the "SARS as scientific mystery" construction was, in effect, to create a climate where investigating the unknown nature of the SARS virus was accomplished in a matter of weeks rather than the months or years it might otherwise have taken.

SARS as a medical epidemic

Although medicine is often treated as if it were little more than an applied science – and it certainly uses all of the resources of the scientific laboratory to accomplish its own intrinsic mission – medicine is ultimately distinct from the scientific discoveries used to support its goals as one of the healing arts. For, whereas the primary focus of the scientific community is on understanding the causative agents of illness, the primary focus of the medical community is on treating the people who are actually ill because of those agents. Thus, for medical practitioners the science of understanding the sources of illness is only a small part of a much larger and more humanistic endeavor: caring for the afflicted in whatever way one can. Especially important in medical practice are all of the individual and social factors related to how patients (and potential patients in the case of a developing epidemic) behave in the face of personal and community illness. Such factors cannot be scientifically controlled.

In the case of SARS, treating the illness as a scientific *mystery* could have had no positive effect for anyone involved directly in the medical dimensions of the epidemic. Medical "mysteries" are far more likely to create panic than to motivate synergistic collective action. After all, there are patients to attend to *now*, and, accordingly, there are therapies or palliatives to administer *immediately*. Whether the physician understands why the patient is manifesting the presenting symptoms or not, something must be done because the patient is *there*. Accordingly, medicine ultimately operates under different constraints than does science, and it needs different constructions of the illnesses it faces in order to guide its medical decision-making in the here and now of immediate patient needs.

The power of competing constructions of an illness to affect individual and collective behavior on a large scale may be seen in how the local and international health care community responded once it determined to classify SARS as a "medical emergency" requiring immediate large scale action and the legitimization of urgent socially disruptive enforcement powers rather than as a localized problem requiring only a localized adaptation of procedures. After all, far fewer people died of SARS worldwide than die of regular pneumonia in Hong Kong every year. And malaria deaths worldwide each year are in the several hundreds of thousands during the same period of time that 299 people died of SARS in Hong Kong. Furthermore, SARS was eliminated as a worldwide medical problem in just four months from the time the first cases began showing up in Hong Kong hospitals.

Classifying SARS as a medical emergency, however, permitted the large scale use of costly medical resources and invited several large scale collective actions (revised hospital procedures concerning gowns and face masks, the creation of new and better isolation wards, quarantines of people exposed to SARS, extensive contact tracings within the community, and so forth) that made the rapid conclusion of the health threat possible. Why do regular pneumonia and malaria, both relatively well understood and treatable diseases, not receive the same urgent medical response as did SARS? Most significantly from a communication perspective is that they are both treated as "endemic" in their locales rather than "epidemic." To classify a disease as "endemic" is to accept that there will always be a number of cases every year because the underlying causes are not remediable. Perhaps it is also to accept that where a disease occurs and who it affects also make a difference to how it is constructed in the hierarchy of medical situations.

Why, then, was SARS constructed as an epidemic disease and therefore as a medical emergency? The features that contributed to turning SARS into a "medical emergency" were such things as its sudden appearance in Hong Kong without warning from mainland officials of the risks, its relatively rapid transmission around the world through air travel, and the fact that a large number of those who were becoming infected and dying were the very health care workers who were treating the SARS patients in the hospital wards. In contrast, malaria is both preventable, and treatable once acquired; but despite its large fatality rate it is not constructed as an *emergency* medical epidemic because (a) it is not a surprise wherever it normally occurs, (b) it is not spreading rapidly to developed countries around the world via routine processes of globalization, and (c) it is not directly transmissible from person to person even in the close quarters provided by routine hospital confinement. Rather, it is acquired indirectly via infected mosquitoes.

In sum, then, if the scientific community may be said to have constructed a vision of SARS as a mystery virus, then the medical community constructed it as a medical emergency. Though the reason patients and medical personnel were getting sick was itself no less a mystery in the early days of the SARS crisis than was the scientific mystery surrounding the nature of the virus itself, the difference to be emphasized here is that the research scientists were concerned primarily with the nature of the viral agent itself, while the medical community was necessarily most intimately involved with the patients who caught the illness and had to be treated. Once the virus had begun afflicting medical personnel in large numbers, SARS could only be constructed as a major medical emergency of large proportions. It was this construction of SARS that permitted the large scale medical responses and the major redirection of medical efforts to proceed as rapidly as they did.

SARS as a public hygiene problem

One of the most remarkable constructions of SARS during the later phases of the crisis was to conceive of the illness as a general public hygiene problem that required a broad cleanup of the way Hong Kong people live. This is a remarkable construction because, as a disease, SARS had a quite specific history that was relatively isolated from the wider-ranging issues in personal hygiene habits or public sanitation behaviors that have long characterized the Hong Kong community. Specifically, the origin of SARS was eventually traced to a form of corona virus (related to the virus that causes the common cold), and its route of transmission into Hong Kong was via a physician visiting from the mainland who stayed at a local hotel. He transmitted the illness to others at the hotel during his very brief visit, and those people eventually infected people in the larger community. As those people also became ill, they not only infected more people within the community but also the medical personnel in the Prince of Wales hospital who treated them, where hygiene and sanitation procedures would be expected to be among the most rigorous. Moreover, once these facts about the origins and transmission of the disease were known, the major way of eliminating the disease involved isolating people exposed to the disease during the possible incubation period so that no further transmission was possible because they were effectively segregated from the community at large. None of this had anything to do with general public hygiene or some broad-based unsanitary conditions in Hong Kong more generally.

However, during the period while details concerning the origins and early transmission of SARS were only slowly becoming known and the disease was far from under control, a particularly large number of cases occurred in a single housing estate known as Amoy Gardens on March 26, 2003. That such a concentrated number of cases could occur in a single, specific residential complex was treated as a symptom of Hong Kong's *general* casualness concerning personal and collective hygiene issues. Suddenly, SARS was conceived as a sign that Hong Kong's attitude toward public hygiene was too casual and lax.

Accordingly, as the community mobilized to fight SARS on many fronts, one of the government's most striking responses was the construction of SARS as a problem in public hygiene and the subsequent development of a public hygiene taskforce known as Team Clean that was originally supervised by the most visible civil servant in Hong Kong, the Chief Secretary of the Civil Service, Mr. Donald Tsang. This taskforce has now become a permanent part of Hong Kong government's health promotion structure, administered under the Home Affairs Department. And Mr. Tsang has been appointed/elected to be the Chief Executive of the Hong Kong SAR until 2012.

Team Clean was officially created on May 5, 2003, with the mission "to establish and promote a sustainable, cross-sectoral approach to improve environmental hygiene in Hong Kong" (Team Clean 2003a, p. 4). The *Interim Report on Measures to Improve Environmental Hygiene in Hong Kong* (Team Clean 2003a), published less than a month after the taskforce was created, stresses several key features of Team Clean's strategic approach: (a) that this must be a community-wide effort and not just a governmental one, (b) that the strategies and accomplishments of Team Clean must be sustainable, and (c) that the Team must break new ground in developing novel approaches to a task that the government had pursued for many years prior to the SARS epidemic.

This last point is really the important one for the theme of this chapter in that the government appears to have understood that earlier efforts "to tackle long-standing problems such as spitting and littering, filthy rear lanes, poorly maintained old tenement buildings, unhygienic food handling practices, smelly restaurant toilets, etc." (Team Clean 2003a, p. 5) had largely failed and that the SARS crisis was really an opportunity to "try to solve old problems" (Team Clean 2003, p. 5) under new (but largely irrelevant) circumstances. The authors of the Interim Report (Team Clean 2003) certainly seem to be fully aware of this linkage.

> A clean and healthy city is built on a community of citizens who observe high standards of hygiene and are keen to keep it that way.
>
> Everything starts with the individual. The outbreak of SARS has heightened public awareness of the important role played by individuals both in maintaining a clean and healthy environment and in preventing the spread of diseases in the community.   (p. 9)

Thus, the goal of the Team Clean taskforce was to take self-conscious advantage of the fear produced by the SARS crisis to promote a much longer term government social goal, namely, producing a generally cleaner Hong Kong. It chose to try to accomplish this more general social purpose by identifying the causes of SARS cases with undesirable public hygiene practices. Here the construction of SARS as a symptom is both conscious and planned to have the effect on social behavior that it subsequently seems to have had. For, as citizens of Hong Kong ourselves, we have not only noticed that the city seems visibly cleaner since SARS, but we have also frequently heard returning visitors remark *without prompting from us* upon how much cleaner the city seems to be compared with their pre-SARS visits. So, more than five years after the founding of Team Clean, and the conscious decision by the government to construct SARS as a symptom requiring a collective "cleanliness response," the results seem to have become quite successful. Linking the interpretive frame to the social goal of inducing greater general cleanliness around Hong Kong appears to have had the desired long term effect that had been sought. Thus, this has been a very successful construction arising from the SARS crisis in the Hong Kong context.

SARS as a government failure

The final construction of SARS we would like to feature ultimately brings us back full circle because this frame accepts that SARS points toward a major government failure to respond adequately to the crisis as it unfolded – a failure that reflects badly on the legitimacy of a government that was not popularly elected and has had little popular support from the beginning of Hong Kong's return to Chinese sovereignty in July 1997.

Even before SARS, Hong Kong's government had been seen as relatively indecisive and far too willing to subordinate the interests of Hong Kong people to those of the mainland leadership's implicit wishes. Among the most troubling of the government's problems in early 2003 concerned what was known locally as "Article 23" legislation. These were somewhat ambiguously worded laws mandated (in principle but not in form or wording) by Article 23 of Hong Kong's mini-constitution (known as "The Basic Law") that would have restricted Hong Kong people's freedoms and which were scheduled to be passed into law on July 8, 2003, without much opportunity for opposition and with little consideration for local opinion and concerns. Then along came SARS, which seemed to have had the effect of limiting the debate even further because of the difficulty of convening public meetings or discussing issues while protected behind surgical masks.

However, about two weeks before the legislation was scheduled to be voted on, Hong Kong was declared free of SARS. On July 1, 2003, a mass protest consisting of over a half million peaceful marchers took to the streets, ostensibly to protest against Article 23 legislation. But, with grassroots citizens having largely constructed SARS as having been worsened by government errors and bungling, the rally size and enthusiasm were surely enhanced by the pent up frustration of a community recently released from the burden of protecting itself from SARS. In the aftermath of the unpredictably large rally, the Article 23 legislation was scrapped, and numerous public officials who had been responsible for actions related to either the legislation or the handling of the government's approach to SARS began resigning over the period of the subsequent twelve months or so.

Accordingly, those who feared that knowledge about SARS would cause social unrest were essentially right! That is, on the political level it has been argued that the handling of the SARS crisis by the government also contributed to community unrest that culminated in anti-government demonstrations in July 2003. For example, DeGolyer (2004) writes that

> The SARS epidemic not only killed 299 people and hospitalized over a thousand in Hong Kong, affected thousands more elsewhere and resulted in worldwide panic; it also directly contributed to and was a major component of the frustration with Chief Executive Tung Chee-hwa's Government that drove half a million people into the streets on 1 July 2003 in the largest demonstrations against a Hong Kong Government since the general strike of the 1920s and the Star Ferry riots of 1966.
>   (p. 135)

Whether the government could have handled SARS much better than it did is certainly not a foregone conclusion (see Chapter 2, this volume, for some discussion of this issue). Undoubtedly, mistakes were made, and a number of post hoc analyses have found considerable room for improvement, so that in the future different approaches would probably be taken should a similar crisis occur. The point to be made here, however, it that once SARS was constructed as an example of "yet another" government failure to safeguard Hong Kong's people's interests, political unrest was almost a foregone conclusion – especially once SARS was linked to other immediate grievances such as Article 23 legislation. When the opportunity to protest became available with the passing of SARS, the July 1 marches provided a necessary catharsis for the entire community. Such is the power of this particular construction of SARS, that even five years later Hong Kong continues to have an annual protest march every first of July, which is now just called the "July 1 Protest" and memorializes whatever it is that Hong Kong people happen to be angry about in government activities and decisions from the previous twelve months. In this view, therefore, the behavioral consequence of constructing SARS as a failure of government action was that it served as a catalyst for social unrest – and perhaps even the beginning of social healing and annual social renewal.

Conclusion

The focus of this chapter has been on the communicative dimensions of Hong Kong's response to the SARS crisis, especially on how various public figures and community groups constructed their understanding (and, therefore, their responses) to the SARS crisis. Its underlying purpose has been to identify a number of social constructions of SARS that influenced how various groups within and around Hong Kong chose to respond to the crisis and its aftermath. In talking about different social constructions of SARS, we have been concerned most specifically with the interpretive frames through which people tried to make sense of the events they were experiencing. We have also indicated how the interpretive frames adopted have consequences for the actions subsequently taken by those individual and groups. This, ultimately, is the lesson to be learned from the present exploration of interpretive frames: it makes a real difference which classifications people use to understand events. Thus, if we wish to understand why people are making the choices they are making, an important place to start is with the language of the frames they have adopted. For, it is these that will signal how they are approaching the decisions they are confronted with as they formulate and implement medical and health related policies.

References and related materials

Brown, S. (2004). The economic impact of SARS. In C. Loh (Ed.), *At the epicentre: Hong Kong and the SARS outbreak* (pp. 179–193). Hong Kong: Hong Kong University Press.

Cao, C. (2004). Chinese scientists were defeated by SARS. In J. Wong & Y. Zheng (Eds.), *The SARS epidemic: Challenges to China's crisis management* (pp. 157–180). Singapore: World Scientific.

Chan, C. L. W. (2003). The social impact of SARS: Sustainable action for the rejuvenation of society. In T. Koh, A. Plant, & E. H. Lee (Eds.), *The new global threat: Severe acute respiratory syndrome and its impacts* (pp. 123–144). Singapore: World Scientific.

Chan-Yeung, M., & Loh, C. (2004). The new coronavirus: In search of the culprit. In C. Loh (Ed.), *At the epicentre: Hong Kong and the SARS outbreak* (pp. 43–54). Hong Kong: Hong Kong University Press.

Chan-Yeung, M. (2004). At the frontline: The medical challenge. In C. Loh (Ed.), *At the epicentre: Hong Kong and the SARS outbreak* (pp. 17–32). Hong Kong: Hong Kong University Press.

Cheng, G. (2004). Healing myself: Diary of a SARS patient and doctor. In C. Loh (Ed.), *At the epicentre: Hong Kong and the SARS outbreak* (pp. 33–41). Hong Kong: Hong Kong University Press.

Chiu, W., & Galbraith, V. (2004). Calendar of events. In C. Loh (Ed.), *At the epicentre: Hong Kong and the SARS outbreak* (pp. xv–xxvii). Hong Kong: Hong Kong University Press.

DeGolyer, M. E. (2004). How the stunning outbreak of disease led to a stunning outbreak of dissent. In C. Loh (Ed.), *At the epicentre: Hong Kong and the SARS outbreak* (pp. 117–138). Hong Kong: Hong Kong University Press.

Gu, X. (2004). Healthcare regime change and the SARS outbreak in China. In J. Wong & Y. Zheng (Eds.), *The SARS epidemic: Challenges to China's crisis management* (pp. 123–155). Singapore: World Scientific.

He, B. (2004). SARS and freedom of the press: Has the Chinese government learnt a lesson? In J. Wong & Y. Zheng (Eds.), *The SARS epidemic: Challenges to China's crisis management* (pp. 181–198). Singapore: World Scientific.

Hospital Authority Review Panel. (September 2003). Report of the Hospital Authority Review Panel on the SARS outbreak. Hong Kong: Hong Kong Hospital Authority.

Koh, T., Plant, A., & Lee, E. H. (2003). (Eds.). *The new global threat: Severe acute respiratory syndrome and its impacts*. Singapore: World Scientific.

Lai, H. (2004). Local management of SARS in China: Guangdong and Beijing. In J. Wong & Y. Zheng (Eds.), *The SARS epidemic: Challenges to China's crisis management* (pp. 77–97). Singapore: World Scientific.

Lau, A. (2004). The numbers trail: What the data tells [sic] us. In C. Loh (Ed.), *At the epicentre: Hong Kong and the SARS outbreak* (pp. 81–94). Hong Kong: Hong Kong University Press.

Lee, L. O.-F. (2003). The impact of SARS on Hong Kong society and culture: Some personal reflections. In T. Koh, A. Plant, & E. H. Lee (Eds.), *The new global threat: Severe acute respiratory syndrome and its impacts* (pp. 93–105). Singapore: World Scientific.

LEGCO Select Committee. (July 2004). Report of the Select Committee to inquire into the handling of the Severe Acute Respiratory Syndrome outbreak by the Government and Hospital Authority. Hong Kong: Hong Kong Legislative Council Printing Office.

Leung, G. M., Hedley, A. J., Lau, E. MC, & Lam, T.-H. (2004). The public health viewpoint. In C. Loh (Ed.), *At the epicentre: Hong Kong and the SARS outbreak* (pp. 55–80). Hong Kong: Hong Kong University Press.

Leung, P. Cheung, & Ooi, E. E. (2003). (Eds.). *SARS wars: Combating the disease*. Singapore: World Scientific.

Loh, C. (2004a). (Ed.). *At the epicentre: Hong Kong and the SARS outbreak*. Hong Kong: Hong Kong University Press.

Loh, C. (2004b). The politics of SARS: The WHO, Hong Kong and Mainland China. In C. Loh (Ed.), *At the epicentre: Hong Kong and the SARS outbreak* (pp. 139–161). Hong Kong: Hong Kong University Press.

Loh, C. (2004c). Lessons learned. In C. Loh (Ed.), *At the epicentre: Hong Kong and the SARS outbreak* (pp. 235–250). Hong Kong: Hong Kong University Press.

Loh, C., & Yip, Y. Y. (2004). SARS and China: Old vs new politics. In C. Loh (Ed.), *At the epicentre: Hong Kong and the SARS outbreak* (pp. 163–177). Hong Kong: Hong Kong University Press.

Loh, C., Galbraith, V., & Chiu, W. (2004). The media and SARS. In C. Loh (Ed.), *At the epicentre: Hong Kong and the SARS outbreak* (pp. 195–214). Hong Kong: Hong Kong University Press.

Loh, C., Welker, J. (2004). SARS and the Hong Kong community. In C. Loh (Ed.), *At the epicentre: Hong Kong and the SARS outbreak* (pp. 215–234). Hong Kong: Hong Kong University Press.

Lorne, F. T. (2003). Will SARS result in a financial crisis? – Differentiating real, transient, and permanent economic effects of a health crisis. In T. Koh, A. Plant, & E. H. Lee (Eds.), *The new global threat: Severe acute respiratory syndrome and its impacts* (pp. 165–170). Singapore: World Scientific.

Ma, N. (2003). SARS and the HKSAR governing crisis. In T. Koh, A. Plant, & E. H. Lee (Eds.), *The new global threat: Severe acute respiratory syndrome and its impacts* (pp. 107–121). Singapore: World Scientific.

Ma, R. (in press). Spread of SARS and war related rumors through new media in China. *Communication Quarterly.*

McNally, C. A. (2003). Baptism by storm: The SARS crisis' imprint on China's new leadership. In T. Koh, A. Plant, & E. H. Lee (Eds.), *The new global threat: Severe acute respiratory syndrome and its impacts* (pp. 31–67). Singapore: World Scientific.

Ng, S. (2004). The mystery of Amoy Gardens. In C. Loh (Ed.), *At the epicentre: Hong Kong and the SARS outbreak* (pp. 95–115). Hong Kong: Hong Kong University Press.

SARS Expert Committee. (October 2003). *SARS in Hong Kong: From experience to action.* Hong Kong: Hong Kong Government.

Seno, A. A., & Reyes, A. Unmasking SARS: Voices from the epicentre. In C. Loh (Ed.), *At the epicentre: Hong Kong and the SARS outbreak* (pp. 1–15). Hong Kong: Hong Kong University Press.

Seow, D. (2003). *SARS: Better understanding and prevention.* Singapore: Unlimited Graphics.

Sung, Y.-W., & Cheung, F. M. (2003). Catching SARS in the HKSAR: Fallout on Economy and Community. In T. Koh, A. Plant, & E. H. Lee (Eds.), *The new global threat: Severe acute respiratory syndrome and its impacts* (pp. 147–162). Singapore: World Scientific.

Tang, S. (2003). Fighting infectious diseases: One mission, many agents. In T. Koh, A. Plant, & E. H. Lee (Eds.), *The new global threat: Severe acute respiratory syndrome and its impacts* (pp. 17–28). Singapore: World Scientific.

Tannen, D. (Ed.). (1993). *Framing in discourse.* New York: Oxford University Press.

Team Clean. (2003a, May). Interim report on measures to improve environmental hygiene in Hong Kong. Hong Kong: Home Affairs Office.

Team Clean. (2003b, August). Report on measures to improve environmental hygiene in Hong Kong. Hong Kong: Home Affairs Office.

Thomson, E., & Yow, C. H. (2004). The Hong Kong SAR Government, civil society and SARS. In J. Wong & Y. Zheng (Eds.), *The SARS epidemic: Challenges to China's crisis management* (pp. 199–220). Singapore: World Scientific.

White, L. T., III. (2003). SARS, anti-populism, and elite lies: Temporary disorders in China. In T. Koh, A. Plant, & E. H. Lee (Eds.), *The new global threat: Severe acute respiratory syndrome and its impacts* (pp. 31–67). Singapore: World Scientific.

Wong, J., & Zheng, Y. (2004). (Eds.). *The SARS epidemic: Challenges to China's crisis management.* Singapore: World Scientific.

Wong, J., Chan, S., & Liang, R. (2004). The impact of SARS on greater China economies. In J. Wong & Y. Zheng (Eds.), *The SARS epidemic: Challenges to China's crisis management* (pp. 11–43). Singapore: World Scientific.

Yuen, K.-Y., & Peiris, M. (2003). Facing the unknowns of SARS in Hong. In T. Koh, A. Plant, & E. H. Lee (Eds.), *The new global threat: Severe acute respiratory syndrome and its impacts* (pp. 173–190). Singapore: World Scientific.

Zheng, Y., & Lye, L. F. (2004). SARS and China's political system. In J. Wong & Y. Zheng (Eds.), *The SARS epidemic: Challenges to China's crisis management* (pp. 45–75). Singapore: World Scientific.

Zou, K. (2004). SARS and the rule of law in China. In J. Wong & Y. Zheng (Eds.), *The SARS epidemic: Challenges to China's crisis management* (pp. 99–122). Singapore: World Scientific.

CHAPTER 2

A hero story without heroes

The Hong Kong government's narratives on SARS

Xiaosui Xiao
Hong Kong Baptist University

This essay addresses a significant question in crisis communication: how should a government perform its role as the official "public narrator" in times of grave disaster? In particular, how should it report its own course of action during and after the crisis? These questions proved to be especially pressing for Hong Kong during the SARS outbreak because the Hong Kong government chose to provide the public with daily reports that highlighted the scientific basis of every step it was taking toward a solution to the crisis. However, in addition to scientifically circumspect information, the public also urgently needed action from the government that could generate stories of bold leadership, bravery in the face of adversity, and heroic accomplishments along the way to the final triumph over SARS. Such narratives were not forthcoming from Hong Kong's official public narrators. Accordingly, this essay examines the government's public statements during the SARS crisis and finds that they failed to provide effective hero narratives to unite the people and stimulate their fighting spirit during the epidemic.

When the World Health Organization declared on June 23, 2003, that Hong Kong was SARS free, everyone assumed that the community healing process would occur rapidly. But it didn't; even today, the citizens of Hong Kong have still not fully recovered from their panic, fear, and resentment concerning the way the Hong Kong government handled the SARS epidemic and its aftermath (Lee 2008; Monks 2008). During the period between March and June 2003, the deadly disease claimed nearly 300 lives and infected more than 1,000 families. In May 2004, anger boiled over after publication of an investigative report by a committee of lawmakers on the government's performance in fighting the SARS epidemic. As a result, the man in charge of health policy in Hong Kong, Dr. Yeoh Eng-kiong, then Secretary for Health, Welfare and Food, was forced to step down, and several other health officials eventually left public service.

After studying the government's public narratives on the SARS epidemic, it is hard to objectively identify any serious problem with the way Hong Kong's officials conducted themselves. For example, did the government narrators fail to report or intentionally cover up the truth of the outbreak? This does not seem to be the case. In fact, the narrators kept the public informed of the numbers of infected patients, the regional locations of infection, the death toll, and so forth on a daily basis from the second day of the outbreak (March 12, 2003). Did, then, the narrators make reckless and ungrounded guesses about the epidemic? Actually, all of the important government updates and reports seem to have had strong scientific grounding. If we blame the official public narrators for not being able to accurately anticipate the spread of SARS, then we appear to be wise after the event. After all, we cannot expect the government to have known beforehand everything about this unprecedented epidemic.

In spite of this, a survey of the editorials and commentaries in Hong Kong's major newspapers reveals an increasingly critical voice against the government as the epidemic intensified (e.g., "Ju buan," 2003, March 25; "Yao daying," March 26; "Chuli weiji," March 27; "Zhengfu ying," March 27; "Fanying," March 28; "Gangfu weihe," March 28; "Granzhi," March 29; "Cuoshi," March 31; "Zhengfu cuoshi," March 31; "Shiqu," April 1; "Tung Chee-hwa," April 2; "Zhengfu shengbing," April 3). The most controversial aspects of the government's response to the SARS crisis centered on whether it was too slow to react to emerging events, and whether it ignored the concerns of the people in the actions it actually did take. It is true that the government narrators appeared to be particularly cautious in predicting the spread of infection. Yet in the light of the scientific narrative frame they were following, such caution is understandable. What, then, has led to the persistent, lingering criticism in Hong Kong that other SARS-affected regions seem to have escaped?

This essay explores these issues from a narrative perspective, arguing that, even though the Hong Kong government may not have committed any serious mistakes in its scientific handling of the new disease, it did have serious problems with its crisis *narration* during the outbreak. The problem with the government's public narratives on SARS lay largely in its overemphasis on "scientificity" as a mode of storytelling. Consequently, it failed to provide effective hero narratives to calm the people and stimulate their fighting spirit. As this essay will show, it is not sufficient to use scientific narration alone to report an official course of action during a grave health disaster. The more that people realize their vulnerability, the more they gravitate toward a central power, which is why most of the Hong Kong media turned to the government as their main source of information during the SARS outbreak. Under this circumstance, the government should have been able to provide great hero narratives, and should have acted as a hero might, to "rescue" its people from unfolding peril.

Accordingly, this case study can help us address a significant question in the field of crisis communication: what role should a government play as a "public narrator" during a grave disaster, whether natural or manmade? Certainly, a government is obliged to inform the public on the state of a situation and the progress of any countermeasures that have been put in place. However, being the official public narrator during a crisis, it will also have to utilize forms of narration that are both politically appropriate and popularly acceptable. In Hong Kong's case, it is truly sad that the government won its battle against SARS in a little less than four months, but failed to leave behind, at least in the minds of many Hong Kong citizens, a good reputation and heroic story of its own actions. The question is why this happened.

To find out, this essay examines the Hong Kong government's SARS crisis narratives as posted on its public website from March through April. These narratives include updates from the Health, Welfare and Food Bureau and the Department of Health, briefings and press releases from government spokespersons, and even statements from Hong Kong's Chief Executive, Mr. Tung Chee-hwa. Reports and comments on these SARS narratives from major news media such as *Apple Daily*, *Oriental Daily*, *Ming Pao*, and *Singtao Daily* were also studied as key references for the government crisis narratives. The essay shows the limitations of scientific narrative in crisis communication and explains how hero narratives can make up for these limitations. It first clarifies the distinction between scientific and heroic narratives and then examines the Hong Kong government's SARS narratives during the peak of the epidemic from the perspective provided by the distinction between scientific and heroic narrative.

Narratives: Scientific versus heroic

Originally theorized only in regard to certain literary forms, narrative is now seen as being almost everywhere, not only in myths, folktales, epic, drama, and novels, but also in popular songs, dance, painting, histories, scientific schema, journal articles, and even our problem-solving activities (see, for example, Andrews et al. 2000; Brooks 1984; Ricoeur 1984; Barthes 1988; Freedman & Combs 1996; Chayat 2006; Winslade & Monk 2007). Narrative can be defined as a chronological arranging of events,[1] and is the way people organize their experiences into

---

1. Shlomith Rimmon-Kenan (1983) is credited with this definition. He defines a story as "a series of events arranged in chronological order" (p. 15).

temporally meaningful episodes (Polkinghorne 1988). Two types of narrative are relevant to this essay: scientific and heroic. Thus, we need to define both types of narrative strategies.

The term *scientific narrative* refers broadly to any narrative that aims at a plain, objective, and factual report of an event or course of action. The words "plain, objective, and factual" here do not imply that scientific narratives simply observe reality in the way that science presumably does; they merely suggest a set of rules that are distinct from the rules that generate more traditional types of narrative. Scientific narrative often focuses on the chronology of the scientific investigation of an event such as SARS, or on the scientific response to such an event. The tracing of an event to its unknown origin, the search for reasonable solutions, and the building of models and theories that are generally applicable constitute the most significant and appealing themes of scientific narrative. The main characters of scientific narrative, whether they be scientists, experts, or political leaders, are often portrayed as firm followers of science, and usually as calm, rational, thoughtful, cautious, meticulously attentive, craving for truth, and caring about the feasibility and benefit of each action that they are going to take.

The term *hero narrative* refers to any narrative that describes a heroic course of action. A hero is a person who "is worshipped and idolized because of his or her morality, excellence and bravery" (O'Sullivan et al. 1994, p. 135).[2] Despite their varied and changing faces in cultural narratives of different time periods, heroes have their commonalities. For example, heroes have to suffer hardships in their adventures to achieve success (Campbell 1968). They also carry a moral or a spiritual mission, and take it as their sacred duty to fight for the weak against the strong but evil ones. This sense of obligation means that they have no hesitation in laying down their lives for people who are suffering, and it gives them the courage to accept responsibility for whatever setback befalls them. In addition, heroes are individuals with potent personalities who hold their followers together because of certain of qualities that make up a great soul. They are seen as resourceful and skillful in problem solving, and they make magnificent contributions to society as a result. Moreover, they are wise and sensible, have a quick insight into people's minds, and have a clear understanding of the needs of the situations they encounter. They thus are able to seize the right time to perform what Redl (1942) calls "the magic of the initiatory act" (cf. Becker 1973, p. 135).

When a crisis is medically-related, such as during the SARS epidemic, the government has the choice of being a scientific narrator, a teller of hero-stories, or both. Both scientific narratives and hero narratives are crucial for people in dire

---

2.   For a recent helpful discussion of the various definitions of hero, see Gibbon (2002).

peril. The more hazardous a situation, the greater the people's need for knowing the truth about their situation. However, they also need hero narratives to help them to maintain a high morale to fight the disaster. For example, a common practice of hero narration during an epidemic is to give public praise and honor to those frontline medical workers who spare no personal sacrifice to save people's lives. But the more important thing for the public to know is that the government is there with the frontline workers to fight for the people and the nation. Thus, the officers often visit infected patients in hospital, an action that is obviously conducted not for medical purposes but, rather, for hero narration and crisis persuasion. Scientific narration represents a rational approach to crisis communication, whereas hero narration represents a motivational approach.

From this introduction, we can see that scientific narrative and heroic narrative represent two very different, if not opposite, approaches to crisis narration – one rational and calm, the other action-oriented and fervent. In spite of this apparent opposition, a government's public narrator should maintain equilibrium between the two, avoiding being either too reserved or too emotional, and striking an adequate balance between the two. Regrettably, during the SARS crisis the Hong Kong government's public narrators were bent on the scientific approach, in spite of the potential grave disaster posed by SARS. It is to the problems caused by this decision that we now turn.

The Hong Kong government's SARS narrative

The deadly SARS virus first struck at Hong Kong's Prince of Wales Hospital on March 11, 2003, infecting more than 20 healthcare workers and causing symptoms of fever and severe respiratory distress. The epidemic reached its peak in April, when many new cases and deaths were reported each day. The disease gradually tailed off after April, until on June 23 the World Health Organization (WHO) removed Hong Kong from the list of infected areas.

Following the initial outbreak at the Prince of Wales Hospital, the government's immediate response was brief and unadorned: the Department of Health was "now investigating into the case" (Press Release [PR], 2003, March 11, 12). It was not until the fourth day, when another wave of infection struck the Pamela Youde Nethersole Eastern Hospital and a private clinic, that the Secretary for Health, Welfare and Food, Dr. Yeoh Eng-kiong, was able to construct a story about the outbreak, which told that some "original patients" had triggered off a cluster of infections in the hospitals, affecting just a few healthcare workers who had had close contact with them. Fortunately, he reported, these patients had not yet had widespread contact with the public that might lead to a large-scale outbreak in the community

(PR, 2003, March 14). A few days later, the public was informed in more detail about this infection story: the suspected cause of the infection was an "unusual" group of atypical pneumonia viruses that were spread through droplets produced by sneezing or coughing. The disease could thus only be transmitted through close contact with infected patients (2003a, March 18; 2003b, March 18).

This version of the infection story, with its scientifically conservative tendency, was quite settling compared with other possible versions that might have been disseminated. The majority of the community, who had not come into contact with the infected parties, could thus rest easy. Dr. Yeoh believed that he was right to reassure the public with this version of the story, because there was no need to induce a widespread panic in the community or to discourage visitors from coming to Hong Kong ("Bingzheng," 2003, March 15). Because early investigations had repeatedly shown that "the clusters of virus focus mainly on healthcare workers and close relatives of the infected patients," can it be said that there was something wrong with this scientifically comforting version (PR, 2003, March 13; March 14; 2003c, March 18; 2003d, March 18)? Probably not, from a scientific narrative viewpoint at any rate.

In the early stage of the outbreak (from March 11 to 26), the official narrators were keen to report the progress of the search for the original patients and to provide scientific updates about the spread of the disease. The searching was a backward investigation of who had been in close contact with whom along the path of the epidemic. The enthusiastic reporting of this search revealed the government's persistent efforts in looking for solid scientific evidence to support its version of the story. On the fourth day of the epidemic, Dr. Yeoh divided the SARS patients into four sub-groups,[3] and then traced each sub-group back to its source (PR, 2003, March 14). This detective work was intriguing in itself, and each sub-group represented a pending case. Who was the culprit? The perfect ending to the search for the government would be to find the four "black hands" that had directly or indirectly touched the four sub-groups of patients. When the traces finally pointed to a suspected index patient (a professor from mainland China) on March 19, then Director of Health, Dr. Margaret Chan (now head of the World Health Organization), immediately announced this happy news as if the government had found a solution to the crisis (2003a, March 19).

However, it was also incumbent upon the government narrators to keep the general public informed of the latest development of the disease. Again, this updating should have been to the government's advantage. If it were indeed the case

---

3.   The first three came from the Prince of Wales Hospital, the Pamela Youde Nethersole Eastern Hospital, and a private clinic. The index patient of the last sub-group was a patient who had been transferred from Vietnam.

that the virus had spread merely through close contact with infected patients, then the daily updates about the epidemic would do nothing more than reproduce the conservative version of the story.

During the early phase of the outbreak, the government's daily report normally started with a general introduction to the developments of the situation (such as new sub-groups that had been found), and then went on to describe the changes in each sub-group, such as any new cases that had been reported, whether confirmed, suspected, in intensive-care, or in the process of recovery. It was desirable to confine the spread of the virus merely to a few hospitals, and then to stop the virus inside the infected bodies before it escaped to kill other people.

Much to their surprise, however, this atypical virus was so atypical that existing medical knowledge and technology could do nothing to stop it from spreading to the community. By March 20, the virus had killed 5 and had been contracted by 145 people. For Dr. Yeoh, however, the infection had not moved far beyond the frame of his earlier narratives: it merely took the form that he least wanted to see, which was that "some of the affected health workers have gone home and carried the disease to their families," thus making what he called "secondary contact" with people who did not have direct contact with the original patients (PR, 2003, March 20).

The official narrators who were keeping track of the developments in case investigation and contact tracing soon found themselves in an embarrassing dilemma, however. The virus had begun plowing through the community, threatening schools and public areas, and the public suddenly realized that they were unexpectedly exposed to the deadly virus. Both the public and the mass media accused the government of inability to contain the disease, and the government's matter-of-fact daily briefings merely served as cynical proof of its ineffectiveness. The investigation and tracing stories were still needed, but they no longer functioned to stabilize an increasingly agitated public.

The government then had to construct more active narratives to calm the public. Following continued demands for a tougher surveillance policy, Hong Kong's Chief Executive declared "war" on SARS in his press conference of March 27. Importantly, the war metaphor set a new frame for future government narratives (PR, 2003a, March 27). "Hong Kong is currently facing its most serious contagious disease threat in [the past] 50 years. The Government will join forces with the community at large to make every effort to win the battle against the disease."

The good news, according to Mr. Tung's story, was that the government for the past 17 days had made substantial progress in the study of the SARS virus. Most important, the government now had "a good grasp of the whole situation" through its ongoing efforts, observations, and investigations. It was thus the critical moment to strike back, as "the preventive measures and surveillance policy put forward by the government are the best in hand" and "the government is confident to win this battle" (PR, 2003a, March 27). Mr. Tung then set down a list of preventive measures and surveillance policies, such as adding SARS to the list of infectious diseases, requiring people who had been in "close contact" with SARS patients to report daily to designated medical centers, suspending all childcare centers, primary, and secondary schools for 9 days, and requiring all visitors to make a health declaration on arrival in Hong Kong.

Mr. Tung's declaration of war actually announced the beginning of what should have become a successful heroic story: the story of the ongoing vigorous and organized fight against SARS. The government was expected to bring this story to a successful conclusion through its heroic course of action. After March 27, the government went further to announce a series of tough actions, which included the isolation of the residents of Block E of the Amoy Gardens housing estate for 10 days, the imposition of restrictions on individual movement in and out of the premises, moving the residents of Block E to quarantine camps on April 1, cleaning and disinfecting every flat of the infected premises between April 7 and 9, the imposition of a "home confinement" quarantine measure for an incubation period of 10 days from April 10 on individuals who had had close family contact with infected patients, and the disclosure of the locations and names of the buildings with confirmed SARS cases on the day of confirmation. Whatever the actual effects of these unusual actions, their announcement and report contributed to the steady unfolding of a war narrative.

Regrettably, a dramatic turnaround in the SARS epidemic did not take place as expected. Given that a number of heroic actions had been taken, the enemy still ran rampant in the community. On April 11, a month after the outbreak of SARS in Hong Kong, the number of confirmed SARS cases had risen to 998 and infection was still on the rise. The government saw the need to retune its war narratives. At this day's press conference, Mr. Tung stated that "the most effective way to avoid the disease is to maintain good personal and public hygiene" (PR, 2003, April 11), hardly a heroic sort of statement.

The continuing spread of SARS seemed to have pushed the government to the end of its narrative resources. For Mr. Tung, it was no longer solely the government's responsibility to fight against the epidemic, but was the obligation of all sectors of society. After April 11, the government rarely initiated any large-scale actions, and the focus of its narratives shifted to activities such as Mr. Tung's visits to hospitals, his commendations to frontline healthcare workers, and the organization of events such as the "Cleaning Hong Kong Action Day."

The construction of scientific narratives

During the SARS crisis, government narrators tried to convey the message that the government was reliable and dependable, and that it was capable of working along "with the community at large to make every effort to win the battle against the disease" (PR, 2003a, March 27). But why should the public listen to the government? The government narrators had to say something more, and tell not just stories, but stories that were trustworthy. This essay argues that the Tung administration basically took a scientific approach and tried to back up its SARS narratives with scientific evidence.

On the very first day of the outbreak at the Prince of Wales Hospital, the government press release gave no details about the incident; but the short statement that the Department of Health was "now investigating into the case" already suggested that the incident, as an unusual medical event, required a great deal of medical expertise and special clinical facilities, and would involve various health specialists (PR, 2003, March 11). Two days later, a government spokesperson reported that the Department of Health was carrying out an investigation in which "question-naires were being used to gather relevant information from staff members for further analysis" (2003, March 12), and that involved the conducting of "laboratory and epidemiological investigation[s] to identify the micro-organism responsible for the outbreak" (2003, March 13). All of these statements indicate that the government was taking a very scientific approach in response to the situation.

On the fourth day, Dr. Yeoh gave the public his first investigation report, from which he derived his story about the infection being limited to hospitals. The report footnoted this story with clinical data.

> The media talked about this atypical pneumonia, saying that there are confirmed cases in the community. This is absolutely right. However, what we are talking about [with] the cases reported these months, we have around 1,500 to 2,000 cases of pneumonia in Hong Kong, and about half are identified to be the bacteria and they are usually easier to treat . . . The other half usually includes a large group of patients with atypical pneumonia. I just want to explain that in any country and any area, there are always cases of pneumonia. . . . In a global sense, since the mode of infection is seasonal, there exists a certain degree of discrepancies. But the distribution is around a 50/50 basically. Actually, this pattern has remained more or less the same for the past few months, and the number that we recorded are similar, so we're not talking about an outbreak of pneumonia in the community. (2003, March 14)

How scientific Dr. Yeoh's argument would sound from an epidemiological standpoint is another story. Nonetheless, the type of argument – using statistical figures and pattern analysis – is what might be expected from a persuasive scientific discourse. As modern scientists would agree, the pattern of statistical distribution usually says more than individual figures. Yeoh's argument was based on his understanding of the pattern or mode of infection, and thus appeared more scientifically sound than the "community outbreak" argument, which seemed to have looked only at individual cases of infection in the community.

March 19 was a day of apparent double blessings for the government. In addition to the Department of Health's celebrated announcement of its breakthrough in tracing the index patients, health experts and microbiologists from the Chinese University of Hong Kong also claimed to have discovered what they believed to be the cause of the SARS infection (PR, 2003b, March 19). The culprit was said to be a virus that belonged to the paramyxoviridae virus family, other members of which include measles and mumps. The successful containment of the disease now seemed well in sight.

By putting the incident under stringent medical surveillance and then placing the suspected virus in a category that was already known to the medical profession, the government was preparing the way for science to deal the whole crisis, which may explain why they did not take action on a grand and spectacular scale before March 27. Health officials must have trusted very much the medical profession in Hong Kong. "With our effective surveillance system and high quality medical and public health services," Dr. Yeoh claimed, "the Hong Kong public and overseas travelers can rest assured that Hong Kong is a safe place" (PR, 2003, March 13). This being the case, it was better to let health officers and medical specialists do their job: people would be fine as long as they followed instructions, such as wearing surgical masks, maintaining good personal and public hygiene, and visiting doctors for the early treatment of respiratory tract infections.

From March 27 onward, the Hong Kong government tried to take a more active, more heroic mode of narration to report its grand battle against SARS. But concern over the scientific legitimacy of the story-telling remained. The official narrators tried to ensure that everything that they said about government decisions and policies would sound scientific and rational.

During a media session on March 27 in which Mr. Tung detailed a set of compulsory measures that were to be introduced against SARS, a serious question was raised: "the Singapore government has suspended classes in schools and began taking isolation measures long ago. Do you think the Hong Kong government is reacting too slowly to take the same measures 17 days after the outbreak?" Mr. Tung replied: "We are working step by step" (PR, 2003b, March 27). Mr. Tung and his health administrator Dr. Yeoh had taken what they believed to be a scientific and reasonable sequence of actions: compulsory measures and a surveillance policy should come into effect after an effective treatment method had been convincingly established. March 27 was perfect timing for the introduction of compulsory measures and a surveillance policy, because the medical profession had just claimed to have found an effective method of treatment, which had been proved to be "80 to 90 per cent effective" (2003b, March 27). It is debatable as to whether this was the right sequence of actions in a crisis such as this, but Mr. Tung seemed to have found sufficient scientific evidence to support the timing of these measures. It must be appreciated that Mr. Tung was still resorting primarily to scientific persuasion to enforce a compulsory policy, although this may not have been the best approach. In contrast, some might argue, Singapore had acted heroically in its own defense. [See, for example, Weber, et al., and Hudson, this volume.]

In a press conference of April 16, the Chief Executive replied to criticism that the authorities had been indecisive in tackling the outbreak: "in fact, we've been very resolute when handling these problems. However, while being decisive and resolute, we need to take careful consideration of every angle and alternative of the problem, and make our progress step by step" (PR, 2003, April, 16). Here, Mr. Tung correctly expressed some of the basic principles of scientific decision-making, as might be found in any introductory textbook on the matter. It is not known whether Mr. Tung had actually practiced these principles in handling the SARS crisis. He did, however, frequently apply them in explaining the process of his administration's decision-making. For example, on March 27 he said: "we've always been observing. After our careful observation we then had a good grasp of the whole situation. Therefore, the preventive measures and surveillance policy put forward by the government were the best" (2003b, March 27). In this explanation, a keen sense of scientific commitment was clearly communicated not only by Mr. Tung's emphasis on the proper act of objective "observation," but also through the strong wording that he used: the government had "always" been observing, until it understood the "whole situation" and could then introduce the "best" measures based on its thorough understanding.

The demand for hero narratives

Despite their scientific rectitude, the government's narratives did not gain popular acceptance. The Hong Kong news media, too, fought for public attention, and their negative and vivid news stories actually spread through the community faster than the SARS virus. In contrast with the government's approach, the media tended to focus on the dark and pessimistic side of the crisis, thereby spreading anti-heroic narratives in the community. By the end of March, the media had successfully constructed a Hong Kong version of *Les Miserables* by spreading terrifying news that informed the public that the virus had captured the whole city, and that SARS had become uncontrollable (e.g., "Ho Siu-wai," 2003, March 25; "Tung Chee-hwa xialing," 2003, March 26). Regrettably, the media's stories of ravage appeared to be more convincing than the government's scientific narratives.

Apparently, being a scientific leader was not enough to manage public fear. In a press conference of March 24, Dr. Yeoh recognized the need for an "adjustment" to the existing policies and strategies on SARS. He believed that the government should act according to two principles: "scientific and clinical experiences" on one side, and "the community's concerns" on the other (PR, 2003, March 24). This suggested that he recognized that science was not the only guide for action in the SARS crisis, and that the government should also accept community concerns and take care of things that originally seemed insignificant from a scientific perspective.

This strategic adjustment implied a new direction for the government narration. When official narrators reported a course of action, they no longer had to indicate whether the actor had taken "careful consideration of every angle and alternative of the problem." For instance, to activate the isolation order on March 31, Dr. Yeoh simply said, "since we cannot identify how the virus was transmitted at the moment, we decided that we needed to have this isolation order to protect the public and the residents" (PR, 2003, March 31). The reason "to protect the public and the residents" was all the government needed to justify its course of action because the safety of the public and the residents was already the community's primary concern at the time.

On March 26, the Chief Executive's Office issued a statement in a heavy tone: "The present situation is serious. It is imperative for us to adopt more effective measures to prevent the virus from further spreading." The government was now "actively considering whether to invoke the Quarantine and Prevention of Disease Ordinance, which empowers the Government to restrict the activities of people having close contact with patients of infectious diseases" (PR, 2003, March 26). This statement on the urgent situation of Hong Kong set a context for the subsequent hero narratives.

After Mr. Tung proclaimed the fight against SARS on the following day, the government narrators became enthusiastic in reporting SARS heroes. Those who were praised ranged from the medical researchers who had been "working days and nights" on arduous investigations (PR, 2003b, March 27), frontline healthcare workers who had "stood fast to their position attending to patients regardless of infection danger" (2003, March 29) and teachers who had "voluntarily stayed behind taking care of school children who had no other places to go during the period of class suspension" (2003, March 29) to those civil servants who had been "relentlessly providing back-up support to our frontline colleagues" (2003, April 7).

Meanwhile, the government belatedly tried to construct a hero story of its own. The scene of the March 27 media session in which Mr. Tung joined with all of his principal officials to declare a war against SARS was an impressive spectacle. Mr. Tung showed much heroic mettle when he pledged to "cut off the path by which the virus spreads" (PR, 2003a, March 27). The tough measures to be taken to "cut off" the path of the virus, such as suspending all kindergartens, primary, and secondary schools, and placing over 1,000 close relatives of the infected patients under close surveillance by the Department of Health, were all heroic undertakings. Although one can always argue that these were simply what the government *had* to do given the circumstances, nonetheless, it is commendable that the government was willing to take on a more active mode of action and to accept greater challenge in adopting the compulsory measures which had not been adopted before.

Unfortunately, this part of the government's role as a hero did not seem to appeal to the public, who criticized it for being "indecisive," "slow to react," and "always lagging behind the times" on the first day that it was determined to act heroically ("Dianxin," 2003, March 28; "Fanying," March 28; "Gangfu weihe," March 28). The problem was that the *public* had called for such heroic measures long before. There is nothing more embarrassing for a hero than realizing that his or her people have clearer foresight about a situation and a better idea about how to react to it. The Tung administration did not seem to be good at learning from its own experiences. Almost every time tougher measures were introduced in the following days, Mr. Tung and his administrators were bombarded with similar charges, such as "slow in reaction," "wavering," and "lacking in foresight," which are not the sorts of qualities associated with a hero (e.g., "Taoda," 2003, April 1; "Guanjian," April 1; "Shiqu," April 1; "Tung Chee-hwa," April 2; "Zhengfu sheng-bing," April 3; "Bingren," April 11).

The criticisms suggest that the Hong Kong government had missed the best opportunity to introduce its hero stories. This essay does not speculate on whether the government should have put forward its anti-SARS measures earlier, but it is certain that the government would have been in a better position to narrate itself into the role of hero if those measures had been announced at an earlier stage in the crisis. As early as March 25, opinion polls suggested that around 60 per cent of Hong Kong citizens recognized the urgent need for school suspension ("Benbao," 2003, March 25). The administration knew very well that if it decided to suspend classes, then it would win "lots of applause," but it preferred to see the community's concern as an emotional reaction and decided to "handle the issue rationally and scientifically" (PR, 2003, March 25).

The situation finally pushed the government into the hero position, but it did not seem interested in seizing this opportunity to make full use of it. Mr. Tung and his administrators were vigorous and decisive in declaring their urgent measures and policies, but when it came to justifying the adoption of these measure and policies, they all withdrew to a prudent and safe scientific discourse. For instance, Dr. Yeoh made a good point in explaining why the government had to issue an isolation order on March 31: "since we cannot identify how the virus was transmitted at the moment, we decided that we needed to have this isolation order to protect the public and the residents." As mentioned earlier, this point was enough by itself to justify the isolation order, but Yeoh perceived that he had not given a full enough explanation of his view, and added another sentence: "obviously, we had done this with our assessment, and the decision has been made after considering all the facts (PR, 2003, March 31).

The second statement immediately altered the nature of the administrative decision. It served little purpose to mention that the decision had been made "considering all the facts," which implies that the safety of the people was merely one of the many factors that the government had taken into serious consideration. Apparently, Dr. Yeoh was trying to re-establish a scientific context of comparing the importance of all of the factors that were involved in the decision to make it appear rational and scientific. The government may well have considered "all the facts" in the course of decision making, and thus the second statement was reasonable from the perspective of scientific narration. However, in terms of hero narrative, this scientific consideration appeared superfluous given that public safety was paramount in the first place.

In another press conference, Dr. Yeoh described how the government decided to invoke the isolation order (PR, 2003, April 10). This time, he did not mention the step of "considering all the facts." Instead, he said: "we've been discussing it for a long time." The goal of this slightly different saying was the same. Dr. Yeoh was trying to mitigate the possible shock that was brought about by the heroic decision by re-projecting the decision as something that resulted from a very rational and scientific process. The implicit message was "true, it was the first time for us to do this. But because we had been discussing it for a long time, it is not a total surprise."

The Hong Kong government earned itself several "first-time" experiences during the SARS crisis: it was the first time that it activated the Quarantine and Prevention of Disease Ordinance, the first time it imposed an isolation order, and the first time it carried out home confinement. These first-time decisions lay at the intersection of science and heroism, and thus the government had the choice of presenting these decisions in a scientific or heroic narrative frame. The government's public narrators kept all of the first-time decisions at a relatively low profile, which is a characteristic of scientific discourse, and used the "first-time" rhetoric in defense of its scientistic policies. The public was frequently told that the government ought to be careful in considering a certain action, because it was the first time that such action had been taken, or because the government had to wait until it was assured of the whole situation, as it had not taken these actions before (2003b, March 27; April 10). First-time action thus became something that had to be managed with great care, rather than being presented as something exciting, something that made history, something done on heroic impulse. On the one hand, this caution can be appreciated given that the situation was one that had never had to be managed before, but on the other, this approach made the heroes invisible. If the initiation of a first-time move has to wait until everything is fully ready, then what do we need heroes for?

From its narrative stance, we can understand why the government was slow to react: it had to take "a long time" to consider and discuss "all the facts." Yet ultimately it still had to say things like "we decided that we needed to have this isolation order to protect the public and the residents," which a hero willing to take whatever action to protect the public and the residents would say. Given this same outcome, why not take the heroic and definitely more humanistic approach from the beginning? Taking a long time to discuss something and considering all of the facts may add meaning to a carefully plotted scientific story, but it turns out to be counterproductive from the perspective of the hero narrative.

Conclusion: Public narratives in times of crisis

Whether through foresight or not, the Hong Kong government defeated SARS in the end, and science had to take much of the credit for the victory. However the cost was heavy, and people believed that many who died in the epidemic were actually victims of the government's failure to respond effectively and in time.

This essay does not comment on the practical aspects of the government's performance during the epidemic. Its strategic approach to crisis narration, however, deserves critical reflection. The government narrators could have been more passionately involved, rather than simply giving scientifically correct and secure speeches. They could have talked sympathetically with the people, rather than criticizing them for being irrational. They could have more actively shown their concern for the people, instead of making empty pledges, such as "we'll make every effort." They could have made use of first-time moves, or initiatory acts, to demonstrate their resolution and determination to fight for the people, and they could have said things such as "that's right, we have never done this before, but if there is a ray of hope then we'll go ahead and strive toward it." This, however, would have required a heroic spirit.

To conclude, there are two major complaints that can be leveled at the Tung administration's response to the SARS epidemic. First, it failed to foresee the developmental trajectory of the epidemic early enough. It is true that among all the countries infected, no government had anticipated the development of the SARS crisis. But the fact that the Singapore government was able to take active and initiatory actions in an earlier period of the epidemic showed that it had better vision about what was going on and how it should respond from its *people's* point of view. This led to the second complaint about the Hong Kong government: it seemed to ignore the public voice demanding heroic actions such as the request for class suspension, despite the fact that the problems that arose revealed the limitations of a scientific narrative.

Scientific narratives tend to be conservative, circumspect, and cautious. Between two possible explanations, scientific narrators are more likely to choose the one that appeals to common sense, unless the other explanation can provide sufficient scientific proof. From this perspective, Dr. Yeoh was right to reject the view that SARS had spread to the community in the early days of the outbreak simply because "there is not sufficient evidence for it." Scientific narrators do not trust foresight and untested intuition: on the contrary, they question and suspect all empirically unverified "knowledge." Furthermore, scientific narrators value "organized observation and careful reasoning," and stress "learn[ing] from the pages of history . . . little by little, slowly line upon line" (Pearson 1892/1991, p. 45). Such a scientific process necessarily takes time, but according to Pearson (1991), "the slowness ought not to dishearten us, for one of the strongest factors of social stability is the inertness, nay, rather active hostility, with which human societies receive all new ideas" (p. 2). Scientific reporters are supposed to dissociate themselves unsentimentally from emotions when giving objective reports, and perhaps it was too much concern for this objective requirement that made the government narrators appear insensitive to the public.

Despite the cloak of science, however, the scientific narrators did not do a very good job of reporting or anticipating the crisis. They had to revise or adjust their stories from time to time in response to the changing situation, which is understandable, but their inaccuracy in assessing the situation, for the author of this essay, was primarily caused by their failure to understand the real needs of the people.

We cannot, of course, put the blame on science; but because of its constraints, scientific narration should not be the single form of public narration used by a government to report on its actions and performance in times of crisis. When facing a fiery ordeal or spiritual challenge, people tend to turn to other forms of narration and appeal to a sense of the heroic. "Times of terror are times of heroism" (Gibbon 2002, p. xxiv; cf. Emerson 1983, p. 380). The SARS crisis was no exception. If there is no time for careful consideration, then a government must respond to deep and powerful impulses such as concern for humanity and justice. Such a government should not need a long time to consider all the facts to figure out precisely what most concerns its people, and it should dare to rescue its people from danger when the urgency arises.

In March and April 2003, the people of Hong Kong urgently needed stories of great government and a heroic course of action to boost their morale and rebuild their confidence. The media portrayed SARS as a monster killer, and the government was left with little choice – it needed to be a hero. However, to become a hero, the government had to demonstrate great concern for its citizens and had to have a particularly strong sense of moral responsibility.

Narration does not simply record an event and a course of action, but also affects the development of the event and the course of action. Had Mr. Tung's administration been determined to perform and then narrate a heroic and daring course of action from the beginning of the epidemic, this painful part of Hong Kong's history might have been written rather differently. Perhaps the fundamental question for the Hong Kong government to reflect upon is not what role it should play in a crisis, but how it should communicate that it cares for its people when the next such crisis occurs.[4]

References

Andrews, M., Schlater, S. D., Squire, C., Treacher, C., & Treacher, A. (Eds.). (2000). *Lines of narrative: Psychological perspectives*. London; New York: Routledge.

Barthes, R. (1988). *The semiotic challenge* (R. Howard, trans.). New York: Hill & Wang.

Becker, E. (1973). *The denial of death*. New York: Free Press.

Benbao mindiao liucheng zancheng tingke [Opinion polls suggests 60 per cent of the citizens want school suspension] (2003, March 25). *Singtao Daily*, p. A2.

Bingren jiashu xu jiazhong geli shitian [Close relatives isolated for 10 days] (2003, April 11). *Ming Pao*, p. A1.

Bingzheng you qianfuqi, liao ranbingzhe yu zheng [Incubation period detected as much more cases are expected] (2003, March 15). *Takong Pao*, p. A1.

Brooks, P. (1984). *Reading for the plot: Design and intention in narrative*. New York: Knopf.

Campbell, J. (1968). *The hero with a thousand faces* (2nd ed.). Princeton, NJ: Princeton University Press. (Original work published 1949).

Carlyle, T. (1983). *On heroes, hero-worship, and the heroic in history*. New York: Chelsea House Publishers. (An edited reprint of the 1908 Everyman's Library edition by J. M. Dent & Sons Ltd. Original work published 1841).

---

4. The arguments in this chapter find some interesting parallels during the foot and mouth crisis in the UK (See Nerlich 2004 and Nerlich, Hamilton & Rowe 2002, for examples).

Chayat, S. (2006). *Life lessons: The art of Jerome Witkin*. Syracuse, NY: Syracuse University Press.

Chuli weiji buneng zhikao kexue [Crisis management cannot rely on science alone] (2003, March 27). *Ming Pao,* A30.

Cuoshi fangyi huangjin shiji, zhengfu ruhe wangyang bulao [Missing the golden chance of fighting the desease, how the government repairs defects] (2003, March 31). *Oriental Daily,* A19.

Emerson, R. W. (1983). *Essays & lectures.* New York: The Library of America.

Dianxin chilai zhaoshu [Typically delayed measures against atypical pneumonia] (2003, March 28). *Apple Daily,* p. A1.

Fanying huanman, zuoshi xianji, zhengfu xu xiqu jiaoxun [Slow in reaction, watching a golden chance slip by, the government should draw a lesson] (2003, March 28). *Oriental Daily,* A31.

Freedman, J., & Combs, G. (1996). *Narrative therapy: The social construction of preferred realities.* New York: Norton.

Gangfu weihe tuole shiqi tian [Why delay 17 days] (2003, March 28). *Hong Kong Economic Times,* A2.

"Gangren zhigang" zhengfu canbai, gangren zijiu shimin chenggong [The government fails to manage, the citizens succeed in surviving] (2003, April 1). *Oriental Daily,* A23.

Giddon, P. H. (2002). *A call to heroism: Renewing America's vision of greatness.* New York: Atlantic Monthly Press.

Guanjian shi fangzhi daijunzhe san bingdu [Stopping virus-carriers from spreading is the key] (2003, April 1). *Wenwei Po,* p. A1.

Guanzhi weixin hezai [Where is the managerial power] (2003, March 29). *The Sun,* D8.

Ho Siu-wai zhongzhao, guanchang konghuang, feiyan gongxian Xianggang [Pneumonia seizes Hong Kong as SARS hits Ho Siu-wai, government in panic] (2003, March 25), *Oriental Daily,* P. A1.

Ju buan wei weisi, zhengfu kangyi houzhibujue [Not prepared for danger in times of terror, the government is slow in fighting the desease] (2003, March 25). *Oriental Daily,* A19.

Lee, E. (2008, February 23). After SARS: Keeping a killer out. *South China Morning Post,* A14.

Leeming, D. A. (1998). *Mythology: The voyage of the hero* (3rd ed.). New York: Oxford University Press.

Monks, S. (2008, February 22). After SARS: Outbreak of fear. *South China Morning Post,* A22.

Nerlich, B. (2004). Towards a cultural understanding of agriculture: The case of the "war" on foot and mouth disease. *Agriculture and Human Values, 21*(1), 15–25.

Nerlich, B., Hamilton, C., & Rowe, V. (2002). Conceptualizing foot and mouth disease: The socio-cultural role of metaphors, frames and narratives. Metaphorik.de, 2, http://www.metaphorik.de/02/nerlich.htm.

O'Sullivan, T., Hartley, J., Saunders, D., Montgomery, M., & Fiske, J. (1994). *Key concepts in communication and cultural studies* (2nd ed). London: Routledge.

Pearson, K. (1991). *The grammar of science.* Bristol: Thoemmes. (Original work published 1892).

Polkinghorne, D. E. (1988). *Narrative knowing and the human sciences.* Albany: State University of New York.

Press Release. (2003, March 11). *DH concerned about PWH case.* Available from Hong Kong Special Administrative Region of the People's Republic of China Web site: www.info.gov.hk/eindex.htm.

Press Release. (2003, March 12). *DH investigating the PWH case.*

Press Release. (2003, March 13). *Surveillance and infection control measures to tackle viral infection cases.*

Press Release. (2003, March 14). *Transcript of Secretary for Health, Welfare and Food.*

Press Release. (2003a, March 18). *Briefings on atypical pneumonia.*

Press Release. (2003b, March 18). *Daily updates on atypical pneumonia from Secretary for Health, Welfare and Food.*

Press Release. (2003c, March 18). *Health Chief briefs consuls general on pneumonia.*

Press Release. (2003d, March 18). *Health Secretary updates on atypical pneumonia.*

Press Release. (2003a, March 19). *Source of pneumonia cases found.*

Press Release. (2003b, March 19). *Virus findings heartening, says Health Secretary.*

Press Release. (2003, March 20). *Transcript of Secretary for Health, Welfare and Food on atypical pneumonia.*

Press Release. (2003, March 24). *Dr. Yeoh Eng-kiong at the press briefing on severe acute respiratory syndrome.*

Press Release. (2003, March 25). *Speech of Prof. Arthur Li Kwok-cheung, Secretary for Education & Manpower Bureau.*

Press Release. (2003, March 26). *Chief Executive's Office issues statement.*

Press Release. (2003a, March 27). *CE announces measures to combat atypical pneumonia.*

Press Release. (2003b, March 27). *Transcript of press conference on atypical pneumonia.*

Press Release. (2003, March 29). *Speech of Prof. Arthur Li Kwok-cheung, Secretary for Education & Manpower Bureau.*

Press Release. (2003, March 31). *Transcript of SHWF's opening statement on the isolation order.*

Press Release. (2003, April 7). *Secretary for the Civil Service writes to all civil servants on combating Atypical Pneumonia.*

Press Release. (2003, April 10). *Transcript of press conference on implementation of home confinement.*

Press Release. (2003, April 11). *Chief Executive's remarks on atypical pneumonia.*

Press Release. (2003, April, 16). *Remarks of CE on atypical pneumonia.*

Raglan, L. (2003). *The hero: A study in tradition, myth, and drama.* Mineola, NY: Dover Publications. (Original work published 1956).

Redl, R. (1942). Group emotion and leadership. *Psychiatry, 5,* 573–596.

Ricoeur, P. (1984). *Time and narrative* (K. McLaughlin & D. Pellauer, trans.). Chicago: University of Chicago Press.

Rimmon-Kenan, S. (1983). *Narrative fiction: Contemporary poetics.* London: Methuen.

Shiqu zixin de haizi [A child lost confidence] (2003, April 1). *Hong Kong Daily News,* c8.

Taoda E-zuo geli, louwang yu ban [Amoy Gardens Block E in quarantine, over half of residents on the run] (2003, April 1). *Ming Pao,* p. A2.

Tung Chee-hwa bu rencuo [Mr. Tung does not admit his fault] (2003, April 2). *Hong Kong Economic Times,* C8.

Tung Chee-hwa xialing buting ke [Mr. Tung says no to class suspension] (2003, March 26). *Apple Daily,* p. A1.

Winslade, J. M., & Monk, G. D. (2007). *Narrative counseling in schools: Powerful and brief.* Thousand Oaks, CA: Corwin Press.

Yao daying feiyan zhanyi, yao zouzai bingdu zhiqian [To win the SARS war, we must run ahead of the virus] (2003, March 26). *Hong Kong Economic Times,* A2.

Zhengfu cuoshi biaoxian liangji [The government has missed a good chance to express itself] (2003, March 31). *Ming Pao,* A25.

Zhengfu shengbing le, heshi cai kangfu [The government is ill, when will it recover] (2003, April 3). *Hong Kong Economic Times,* A20.

Zhengfu ying cai geng yange cuoshi fang bingdu kuosan [The government should take tougher measures to contain the spread of virus] (2003, March 27). *Takung Pao,* A15.

CHAPTER 3

"SARS" versus "atypical pneumonia"
Inconsistencies in Hong Kong's public health warnings and disease-prevention campaign

Gwendolyn Gong and Sam Dragga
Chinese University of Hong Kong / Texas Tech University

When Hong Kong first reported cases of SARS, the government developed a public health campaign to warn and educate the local community and international travelers about the highly-contagious disease. Unfortunately, concern that the similarity of the acronyms for the Hong Kong Special Administrative Region (Hong Kong *SAR*) and the illness (*SARS*) would have negative political and economic impact on the territory appears to have led Hong Kong officials to use the term *atypical pneumonia* interchangeably with *SARS*, the official name coined for the illness by the World Health Organization, long after it was appropriate to do so. This errant usage probably resulted in inconsistent and misleading public health information, late quarantine policy, inadequate safety measures, and higher than necessary infection and death rates. The lessons of Hong Kong's tragic experience are familiar: words are important, words have consequences, and words are ethical choices that can make a difference in how people respond to the events that are labeled by them.

In November 2002, a highly contagious "mystery" illness first appeared in China's Guangdong Province, which shares a border with Hong Kong. However, as one clinical review notes, the outbreak in southern China "was not widely publicized, and the condition remained isolated to China for the next 3 months" (Sampath-kumar, Temesgen, Smith, & Thompson 2003, p. 882).

This situation changed on February 21, 2003, when a doctor from Guangdong Province who had been treating patients contracted the virus and then traveled to Hong Kong to visit relatives. This mainland doctor stayed on the ninth floor of Hong Kong's Metropole Hotel, was hospitalized at the Kwong Wah Hospital on February 22, and died of respiratory failure on March 4. This doctor was the "Hong Kong index patient" who spread the disease from southern China, directly infecting two family members and four health care workers in Hong Kong. In fact, March 3, the day before the index patient died, is considered in government reports as the official date when the epidemic began in Hong Kong.

The illness presented symptoms similar to those found in persons afflicted with typical pneumonia (i.e., a bacterial infection in the lungs), but unlike typical pneumonia, this mysterious sickness was viral and thus did not respond to the antibiotics normally prescribed. Therefore, the mystery disease was, at first, classified as "atypical pneumonia," which is a general designation used in Hong Kong and China for labeling a wide variety of routine viral pneumonias that frequently require some period of patient hospital care but which do not usually necessitate special staff precautions or community alerts. But this one was different because of its highly contagious and deadly nature, so much so that on March 15, the World Health Organization (WHO) gave the new virus the official descriptive tag: *Severe Acute Respiratory Syndrome* or *SARS* to indicate its unique status among superficially similar respiratory diseases. Moreover, special procedures were promulgated by health authorities for handling the disease in both the clinical and community setting.

Surprisingly, the term was not "adopted" by the HKSAR government until March 27 – a lapse of 12 days. For, upon hearing of the WHO's name for the disease, a number of Hong Kong's politicians, health officials, tourism chiefs, and business officials mobilized; they did not want the virus to be linked with the Hong Kong **SAR** (the SAR denotes Hong Kong as a Special Administrative Region of China). For politically- and economically-motivated reasons, then, Hong Kong's government opted to substitute or use both terms (i.e., *SARS* and *atypical pneumonia*) in the majority of their public health messages.

The purpose of this chapter is to examine selected public health texts produced by the government during the SARS epidemic in order to analyze the political and economic considerations that appear to have influenced Hong Kong's public health officials to use two different terms for the infectious disease: *SARS* and *atypical pneumonia*. The analysis of the inaccurate use of these two terms reveals how the government's concern about its image came in conflict with the clarity of its health communication messages during this epidemic, calling into question its judgment concerning where its sense of ethical responsibility rested.

Data set analyzed

At the time of the SARS outbreak, Dr. E. K. Yeoh was the Secretary for the Health, Welfare and Food Bureau, the chief politically-appointed officer responsible for the government's handling of the SARS outbreak in Hong Kong. Dr. Yeoh oversaw five departments, including the Department of Health, directed by Dr. Margaret

Chan, and Hong Kong's Hospital Authority, directed by Dr. William Ho. For the most part, the Department of Health was responsible for developing a local public health campaign about SARS – a multimedia and multilingual communication initiative – to inform Hong Kong's international citizens and visitors about the health crisis situation. The Hospital Authority was in charge of coordinating the campaign for health professionals, hospitals, and emergency wards. Accordingly, administrative personnel under Dr. Yeoh's direct supervision created a wealth of information in a variety of formats in a short span of time; so we have a large data set available to analyze. These include:

- Government websites
- FAQ fact sheets
- Announcements (e.g., infection and death rates, government reports on "hot-spot" housing estates, list of buildings with confirmed SARS cases, schedule for talks about SARS)
- Health advice for specific audiences (i.e., the community, public transport professionals, medical and health care professionals, travelers, educators and students)
- Publicity materials (leaflets focusing on hygiene, disease prevention, and health advice and guidelines, posters, TV and radio announcements, and downloadable PowerPoint presentations)
- News reports and editorial analyses
- Post-SARS hearings and reports

During the crisis, the data in these sources had to be constantly updated and re-issued, with copies oftentimes forwarded in special reports to the World Health Organization and the Center for Disease Control. To keep track of a developing epidemic and simultaneously provide both health education and current information to the public was a daunting task (cf. Arguin, Navin, Steele, Weld, & Kozarsky 2004). However, it provides a rich resource to analyze. Accordingly, we collected data from all of these sources to see how the official government sources were handling their public health messages over time.

What we found from our analysis was that, even after March 27, 2003, when the Hong Kong government officially accepted the WHO's name for the new disease, the government remained at great pains to avoid using the SARS acronym in its publications and announcements. Moreover, more often than not, it did not use the WHO's official four-word name for it either. Rather, until mid-May it almost uniformly defaulted back to the more medically innocuous and politically-expedient *atypical pneumonia* label. This had the effect of essentially hiding the true nature of the epidemic from the public and government critics by substituting a euphemistic label designating a relatively routine set of illnesses for the special purpose label created by the WHO to signal the exceptional dangers of the new disease.

Chronology of SARS health communication information

To illustrate the point that Hong Kong's public health officials were loathe to adopt the WHO's term in their public messages, the following paragraphs detail a number of cases in which Hong Kong's Department of Health tried to avoid using the official designation of Severe Acute Respiratory Syndrome (and especially the acronym SARS) in its advisories to the public.

For example, on March 20, a medical advisory to doctors from Hong Kong's Department of Health was issued (retrieved May 12, 2003, www.info.gov.hk/dh). Titled "Letter to Doctors on Atypical Pneumonia Outbreak in Hong Kong," the advisory ignores the official WHO designation for the disease and refers exclusively to *atypical pneumonia*. The advisory details symptoms of the disease (e.g., fever, malaise, chills) in 31 of 145 known cases and summarizes the findings of available epidemiological investigations.

On March 24, on the official website of the Department of Health, prevention information aimed at the general public refers to both atypical pneumonia and Severe Acute Respiratory Syndrome, but it constructs its discourse contrastively, as though the two diseases were different:

> The World Health Organization recently received reports of "Severe Acute Respiratory Syndrome" in various parts of the world. In Hong Kong, a number of health care workers and other people have also been affected by atypical pneumonia. ("Prevention of Atypical Pneumonia," retrieved May 12, 2003, www.info.gov.hk/dh)

The implication here is that while Severe Acute Respiratory Syndrome might be occurring outside Hong Kong, inside Hong Kong the worry is atypical pneumonia – a different disease. The information on this page subsequently proceeds to differentiate typical from atypical pneumonia (bacterial versus viral origins) and offers guidelines for avoiding infection. Only once is Severe Acute Respiratory Syndrome mentioned: the acronym of SARS is never used.

Two days later, on March 26, a page on the official website of the Department of Health aimed at tourists is still referring to the disease as atypical pneumonia but acknowledges that this is the same disease that WHO has identified as Severe Acute Respiratory Syndrome:

> The World Health Organization (WHO) recently received reports of Severe Acute Respiratory Syndrome, commonly known as atypical pneumonia, in various parts of the world. ("Information for Visitors to Hong Kong," retrieved May 12, 2003, www.info.gov.hk/dh)

In this passage, the Department of Health is insisting, through the parenthetically inserted "commonly known as atypical pneumonia," that the two diseases are the same and that the *atypical pneumonia* label is the more widely used and better understood designation for the disease. The SARS acronym, however, is never used. Furthermore, the page is filled with general information designed to comfort tourists (e.g., praise of Hong Kong's "world-class medical services and facilities"), including the claim that "Hong Kong is working closely with the WHO" to avert a possible epidemic. Thus, the message to tourists is that nothing special is going on in Hong Kong and that it is as safe to travel there as it has always been.

Then, in a new medical advisory to doctors on March 27 – issued twelve days after the WHO identified the disease as SARS – Hong Kong's Director of Health drops all mention of *atypical pneumonia* and identifies the disease as Severe Acute Respiratory Syndrome (see Figure 1). The SARS acronym, however, is still avoided. Importantly, however, with the change in label from atypical pneumonia to Severe Acute Respiratory Syndrome also comes a significant change in how people contracting the desease may be treated. For the letter explains that **individuals with the disease are subject to quarantine and cases of infection must be reported by all medical practitioners to the Director of Health.** Thus, the change in terminology is significant both practically and theoretically in that the different categorical label for the disease permits a different set of community health procedures to be legally implemented: reporting is required and quarantining is allowed.

In spite of the importance of the change in public health policies signaled in the message to physicians on March 27, a press release from the Department of Health two days later (March 29) urges public participation in a "Household Cleaning Day" on March 30 in a community effort at "containing the spread of atypical pneumonia" (retrieved May 12, 2003, www.info.gov.hk/dh). No mention is made of either Severe Acute Respiratory Syndrome or SARS. So, the government has essentially retreated from its new designation, at least when addressing the general public.

A press release issued on March 31 regarding the imposition of a 10-day quarantine on the residents of one apartment building in the Amoy Gardens housing complex (the residents would later be evacuated) is equally ambiguous. The isolation of the residents was designed "to prevent the spread of Severe Acute Respiratory Syndrome (commonly known as atypical pneumonia)" – indicating a continuing resistance to the WHO's designation as foreign and technical but not

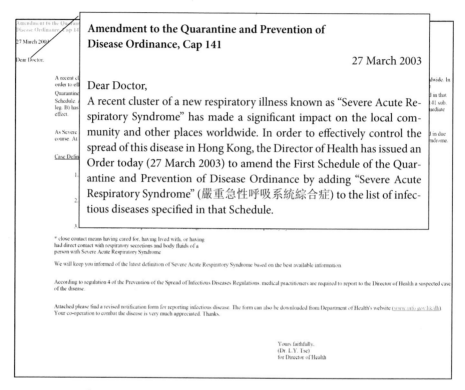

Figure 1. March 27, Amendment to the Quarantine and Prevention of Disease Ordinance (SOURCE: www.info.gov.hk/dh, retrieved May 12, 2003)

medically significant in determining the Department's quarantine policies or actions. The acronym of SARS is never used (see Figure 2).

The transcript of the opening statement by the Secretary for Health, Welfare and Food, Dr E. K. Yeoh, at the press briefing on the isolation order, contributes to the confusion:

> As you know we had this outbreak of what we called atypical pneumonia, which has been called severe acute respiratory syndrome. (Press Release on Transcript of Secretary's Statement, retrieved May 12, 2003, from www.info.gov.hk)

In addition to continuing the tendency to subordinate the new disease to the more benign category of *atypical pneumonia*, it is especially important to note in this passage the use of passive voice, which leaves the origin of the "Severe Acute Respiratory Syndrome" label agentless and anonymous. By omitting mention of the World Health Organization in this sentence, Dr. Yeoh appears to be trying to make the two designations of the disease equally official and authoritative. The

Press Rele

✉ **Email**

Director of Heal

****

> Director of Health, Dr Margaret Chan, has ordered Block E of Amoy Garden in Ngau Tau Kok, Kowloon Bay, to be isolated for a period of 10 days starting from 6 am this morning (March 31) to prevent the spread of Severe Acute Respiratory Syndrome (commonly known as atypical pneumonia), a Government spokesman said.

Director of Health, Dr Margaret Chan, has ordered Block E of Amoy Garden in Ngau Tau Kok, Kowloon Bay, to be isolated for a period of 10 days starting from 6 am this morning (March 31) to prevent the spread of Severe Acute Respiratory Syndrome (commonly known as atypical pneumonia), a Government spokesman said.

The decision was taken because of the continued steep rise in the number of cases of infection in the building in the past few days.

The order, designed to protect the health of residents and the community as a whole, was issued under the authority granted under Section 24 of the Prevention of the Spread of Infectious Diseases Regulations, Cap. 141.

The order requires residents of Block E of Amoy Garden to remain in their flats until midnight on April 9.

During the isolation period, no one will be allowed to enter or leave the premises without express permission in writing of a health officer.

Medical personnel from the Department of Health will visit residents' homes to conduct health inspections for them. Residents will be provided three meals a day free of charge. They will also receive help and advice to conduct thorough cleansing and disinfection of their flats. Staff of the Home Affairs Department will be briefing residents on the detailed arrangements to take care of their daily needs.

"We do understand that the measures that we have now taken will cause residents great inconvenience. But because of the very special circumstances that we now face, we have no choice but resort to this exceptional measure and we sincerely ask for residents' forbearance, understanding and support in joining the community's fight against this disease." the spokesman said.

End/Monday, March 31, 2003

Figure 2. March 31, Press Release on Isolation Order (SOURCE: www.info.gov.hk/dh, retrieved May 12, 2003)

audience for such a statement could easily conclude that the source of the new label was insignificant. We also note that the SARS acronym is still never used in spite of its relevance to the public actions that are being discussed at the press briefing.

While the Department of Health was still at pains to avoid or minimize the official WHO designation for the disease, a press release the same day by Hong Kong's Social Welfare Department reveals no such misgivings. This notice, titled "Emergency Financial Assistance for people affected by SARS," is the first time we could identify a unit of the Hong Kong government using the SARS acronym to discuss the growing epidemic – **16 days after the WHO adopted its official designation** (retrieved May 12, 2003, www.info.gov.hk). No mention is included here of *atypical pneumonia,* and the relationship of the full name of the disease to the acronym is made explicit: "patients suffering from Severe Acute Respiratory Syndrome (SARS)." The following day (April 1), however, on the official website of the Department of Health (retrieved May 12, 2003, www.info.gov.hk/dh), a page explaining ways to avoid infection continues to identify the disease only as *atypical pneumonia.* Neither the four-word title nor the acronym of SARS is used.

Six days later, on April 7, using materials issued by the Department of Food and Environmental Hygiene, a page on the official website of the Department of Health still carries the title "Atypical Pneumonia: Guidelines on Inspection and Disinfection of Common Parts of Buildings" and avoids all mention of Severe Acute Respiratory Syndrome or SARS. Similarly, on April 9, using information issued by Hong Kong's Department of Labour, a page on the official website of the Department of Health carries the title "Atypical Pneumonia: Guidelines for Employers and Employees," but mentions severe acute respiratory syndrome and claims its relationship to atypical pneumonia:

> Severe acute respiratory syndrome is an acute respiratory infection that has been reported in a number of places, including Hong Kong. It is a form of atypical pneumonia caused by a new agent. ("Guidelines for Employers and Employees," retrieved May 12, 2003, www.info.gov.hk/dh)

The words *severe acute respiratory syndrome* are used five times on the page but without initial capital letters (unless at the beginning of a sentence), thus disrupting recognition of the SARS acronym. The following claim is also offered on the page:

> The Hong Kong SAR Government is joining hands with the World Health Organisation to combat the disease on all fronts. ("Guidelines for Employers and Employees," retrieved May 12, 2003, www.info.gov.hk/dh)

The inclusion of the SAR acronym in this passage (Special Administrative Region), would make it especially politic for Hong Kong officials to avoid juxtaposing the almost identical acronym of the disease.

By April 22, the Health, Welfare and Food Bureau of the Department of Health finally issues a "SARS Bulletin" that summarizes cases of "Severe Acute Respiratory Syndrome (SARS)" and uses the acronym consistently and in grammatically flexible ways as both a noun and adjective (e.g., SARS cases, SARS patients), indicating its genuine adoption as a valid word of the language. No mention is made of atypical pneumonia. The title of "Special Administrative Region" is used – in the same paragraph as two occurrences of the SARS acronym – but the SAR acronym for Hong Kong is never displayed. Nevertheless, the same day, a page on the website aimed at boys and girls (or so the illustrations indicate) carries the title "Prevent Atypical Pneumonia: For Health to be Bright/Get the Hygiene Right" and makes no mention of Severe Acute Respiratory Syndrome or SARS (retrieved May 12, 2003, www.info.gov.hk/dh).

However, on April 25, the words *Atypical Pneumonia* (newly capitalized in all occurrences) are the subject of "A Reminder for Parents" that offers guidelines for preventing infection of children (see Figure 3). The words *Severe Acute Respira-*

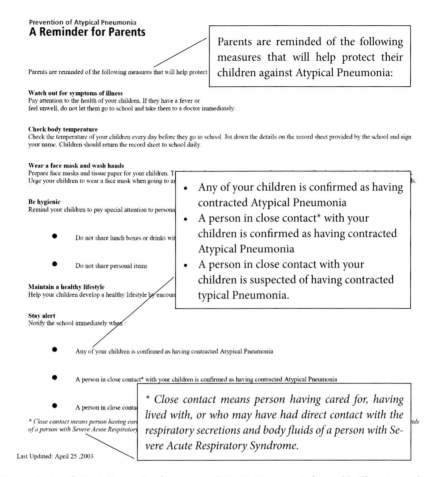

Figure 3. April 25, A Reminder for Parents (SOURCE: www.info.gov.hk/dh, retrieved May 12, 2003)

tory Syndrome are used only once in a note, in italics, at the bottom of the page. The familiar SARS acronym is never used.

On May 2, a guidebook issued by Hong Kong's Department of Justice and a corresponding page on its official website try to summarize "the most relevant laws that relate to the control of atypical pneumonia." Severe Acute Respiratory Syndrome is mentioned (always buried in lists and paragraphs), but the SARS acronym is never used (see "A Summary of Hong Kong's Hygiene Laws," http://www.info.gov.hk/dh).

On May 11, almost a full two months after the WHO identified the disease as Severe Acute Respiratory Syndrome or SARS, Hong Kong's Department of Health is still quibbling. While a public notice is titled "Travel Advisory on Atypical

Pneumonia," it nevertheless adopts the international designation of the disease as well as the acronym that Hong Kong officials have been resisting. It is noteworthy – and possibly daring – that both *SARS* and *Hong Kong SAR* are used in the same paragraph. The usage, however, is still inconsistent: for example "All out-bound and in-bound travelers should be aware of main symptoms and signs of Severe Acute Respiratory Syndrome (SARS)" but "It is prudent for tourists to adopt the following precautionary measures to prevent atypical pneumonia." Inconsistent or divided usage is also evident in two tables of quantitative information issued on the same day. The information given to the public is titled "Latest Figures on Severe Acute Respiratory Syndrome" with no mention of atypical pneumonia, while the same information given to schools in the "Daily AP Bulletin for Schools" is identified as "Overall figures of confirmed atypical pneumonia cases" with no mention of Severe Acute Respiratory Syndrome or SARS (see tables at http://www.info.gov.hk/dh).

Political and economic concerns: What's in a name?

The previous examples illustrate that the Hong Kong government was issuing confusing and misleading information about the SARS epidemic long after the WHO gave the disease its own name for the very purpose of separating it from the general category of atypical pneumonias with which it was first identified. Its ease of transmission and particular virulence meant that SARS was not a simple "atypical" pneumonia, but a truly new disease. So the public, tourists, and even at times the health care community were influenced to misunderstand and under regard the dangers posed by SARS during the early phase of the epidemic.

However, public confusion is not really the most important consequence of the government's lexical choices from a communication point of view. For those choices also had clear implications for how quickly and flexibly the government was able to respond to the spreading epidemic and how willing the public might have been to accept the more drastic measures the new designation would have permitted, such as the imposition of quarantine orders and forced relocations away from infected population areas. As noted earlier, the WHO issued an advisory on March 15, referring to the virus for the first time as *Severe Acute Respiratory Syndrome* or *SARS* – a name whose acronym was considered by many locally to be "a cruel pun" on the fact that the HKSAR had been the first to officially report the virus. But the WHO's designation also meant that SARS was being identified as a new illness caused by a new infectious agent that required new and more aggressive community responses.

Therefore, rather than privileging concerns about the potential damage caused by the WHO's unintended pun, officials should, of course, have kept public safety as their central objective. For, to have adopted the WHO's label and definition would have permitted the Hong Kong health authorities to begin quarantining suspected SARS patients immediately under the WHO rules for virulently contagious diseases. By rejecting the WHO designation for 12 days, the government was prevented from taking actions that could have slowed the spread of the disease during a critical period when it might have been more easily controlled.

Did government authorities know that their lexical choices were promoting an inaccurate picture of the disease as it spread throughout the community? Although this would be difficult to prove definitively, there is a piece of corroborating evidence that indicates the government and Dr. Yeoh were keenly aware of the difference between SARS and atypical pneumonia. In investigative hearings on the SARS outbreak by Hong Kong's Legislative Council, the government was found to have knowingly used these two terms in fuzzy, confusing, and misleading ways. For example, Dr. Yeoh's testimony revealed the rhetorical skill he had demonstrated during a crucial press conference conducted 10 days after Hong Kong reported its first case of SARS to the WHO. As reported in the *South China Morning Post* (Moy 2004),

> The health chief yesterday defended his remarks last March that there was no outbreak of Sars [sic] in the community, saying reporters had asked the wrong question.
>
> Secretary of Health and Welfare Yeoh Eng-kiong told a Legco inquiry panel that he was responding to questions about atypical pneumonia on March 14 last year, rather than severe acute respiratory syndrome.
>
> He insisted he did not hide the Sars outbreak from the public.
>
> "When you talk about atypical pneumonia, it is a generic description for a group of diseases; it is not a very specific term. Even now the people in the medical sector have difficulties in defining it," he told reporters after the panel meeting.
>
> "So on the 14th, I described the situation of pneumonia in Hong Kong. I described how many cases we saw and that the information provided to me by the Hospital Authority and the Department of Health showed no increase in those cases.
>
> "So, I was describing the whole phenomenon of atypical pneumonia."
>
> (p. A4)

Dr. Yeoh clearly knew the difference between SARS and the general term, *atypical pneumonia*, cleverly shifting blame for not addressing the incidence of the "new, mysterious virus" in Hong Kong during the press conference because reporters queried him about atypical pneumonia instead. It is important to note that this politician and medical professional did not attempt to clarify the meaning (and thus the inappropriate use) of the "atypical pneumonia" label to the media; this was a missed opportunity, early on, to educate members of the press. From Dr. Yeoh's testimony, however, it seems clear that his intention was not to educate or clarify medical information to the press; on the contrary, his purpose seemed to be to "spin" – to mislead and misdirect.

In hindsight, we can see that this kind of rhetorical spin had even more disastrous consequences. Because of the misleading use of terminology, quarantine measures that might have reduced the early spread of the disease were seriously delayed. This consequence came to light during a Legislative Council SARS hearing, where Dr. Margaret Chan confirmed what many in the community had suspected:

> There was a 12-day delay in adding Sars [sic] to the list of diseases for which people could be forced into quarantine because Hong Kong's health chief was opposed to calling the illness Sars and had doubts about its definition. . . .
>
> Secretary for Health, Welfare and Food Yeoh Eng-kiong was not happy that the name – coined by the World Health Organisation on March 15 – sounded like the acronym for the special administrative region, Margaret Chan Fung Fu-chung told a Legco committee on Sars.
>
> Dr. Yeoh had suggested the word "acute" be dropped so that the disease would be known as "SRS" – for severe respiratory syndrome, instead of Sars for severe acute respiratory syndrome.
>
> "I had no arguments with him. I only said that there was no way for us to argue with the WHO."
>
> Dr. Chan said implementing quarantine and isolation orders in an infected area such as Hong Kong would have meant isolating a huge number of people.
>
> She said top-level deliberations by the Sars Steering Committee – chaired by Chief Executive Tung Chee-hwa to guide the government's response to the outbreak – over the definition of Sars led to a 12-day delay in adding Sars to the list of quarantinable diseases.
>
> The quarantine ordinance was finally invoked on March 27 to include Sars.
>
> Dr. Chan said if the WHO definition had been accepted immediately, the ordinance could have been in place on March 16 or 17.   (Benitez 2004, p. A4)

Dr. Chan's testimony exposed to the public what dire consequences the government's medical word play had yielded.

The price of the rhetorical "spinning"

There is no doubt that SARS took a terrible toll on Hong Kong. In bare statistical terms, 299 people died, including eight healthcare workers; another 1,221 people caught the disease, but recovered. However, even among the patients who recovered, chronic long term health problems often continue. For example, 158 SARS survivors in Hong Kong have already been diagnosed with avascular necrosis, a disease that stops blood flow to the bones. It is believed that patients developed avascular necrosis because of the heavy doses of corticosteroids used to treat SARS. This drug therapy was considered the only treatment that could "fight" SARS, despite also causing bone disease in patients. Moreover, as recently as August 2004, new reports indicated that there were another 200 patients who are "either too young to be scanned since their bones have not fully developed, or have yet to be located by the Hospital Authority" (Wu 2004, p. A16). Other patients who were misdiagnosed with SARS were also treated with corticosteroid drugs, and some of them are now also suffering from the crippling bone disease.

It is impossible to know for certain, of course, that the government's reluctance to accept the WHO's label for SARS, and its continued ambivalence in using the term once it was finally officially accepted, contributed substantially to these high numbers and severe consequences, though it seems a reasonable conclusion from Dr. Chan's observation that the quarantine ordinance could have been applied to SARS much earlier had the designation been quickly adopted and unambiguously embraced in government thinking and public communications. Things were certainly made worse, though we cannot quantify by how much.

However, we can identify other kinds of costs resulting from the government's tendency toward rhetorical spinning. For example, three of the public officials centrally involved in the dissemination of public health information eventually resigned under pressure, and a fourth left Hong Kong to join the WHO. In particular, Health minister Dr. Yeoh Eng-kiong resigned on July 7, 2004, three days after a critical Legislative Council Select Committee report blamed him for mishandling the SARS outbreak (Benitez & Lee 2004, p. A1); Hospital Authority chair Dr. Leong Che-hung resigned on July 8, 2004 (Benitez, Lee, & Lo 2004, p. A1); and Hospital Authority executive Dr. Ko Wing-man resigned on August 31, 2004 (Wong 2004, p. C4). Only former Director of the Health Department, Dr. Margaret Chan Fung Fu-chun, survived the criticism arising from the crisis. Late in 2003, she became the WHO's Director of the Department for Protection of the Human Environment; in 2005 she was appointed as its Director for Communicable Diseases Surveillance and Response, as well as being the Representative of the Director-General for Pandemic Influenza. In November 2006 she became the Director-General of the WHO.

Yet another kind of cost produced by the misguided attempt at spin control is that several investigative committees were formed and numerous legislative hearings were held, resulting in a number of analytical and critical government reports. For example, the SARS Expert Committee was created as an independent Commission of Inquiry, appointed by Hong Kong's Legislative Council, on May 28, 2003 (Chiu & Galbraith 2004, p. xxvii). It published its report on October 2, 2003. This report focuses on lessons learnt from the epidemic, but does not pin-point blame or responsibility. Shortly thereafter, on October 29, 2003, the Legislative Council appointed a Select Committee to look into how the SARS outbreak was handled by the Government and the Hospital Authority, and to judge the performance of the officers at policy-making and management levels for accountability purposes (Legislative Council Select Committee 2004, p. 2). The Select Committee published their report on July 7, 2004. It was after this report appeared that the public officials mentioned in the previous paragraph began to resign in rapid succession.

Conclusion

This chapter has investigated discourse produced by Hong Kong government officials during a critical period in the development of the SARS epidemic. It has focused particularly on the tendency of those officials to speak and write ambiguously when labeling the disease, even after the WHO gave the disease its own special name and status. Local officials apparently made that choice because the WHO's label appeared to echo Hong Kong's full name as a Special Administrative Region (SAR) of the People's Republic of China. It was argued that the tendency to communicate ambivalently led those same officials to delay in treating SARS as a quarantine-invoking illness, and that more people became ill than otherwise might have because of the delay in accepting the WHO's label and the corresponding reclassification of its seriousness. Finally, the chapter has pointed out some of the negative social and political consequences that arose in the aftermath of the SARS crisis, consequences that seem fairly directly attributable to the Hong Kong government's lexical choices when talking about the disease.

Thus, while the lessons from Hong Kong's experience with SARS are several, for scholars interested in the rhetoric of public health communication, the most important may be tragically familiar: words are important, words have consequences, words are ethical choices. And sometimes words are a matter of life and death.

References

Arguin, P. M., Navin, A. W., Steele, S. F., Weld, L. H., & Kozarsky, P. E. (2004, February). Health communication during SARS. *Emerging Diseases, 10*, 377–380.

Benitez, M. A. (2004, January 14). Quarantine delayed for days by row over name. *South China Morning Post*, p. A4.

Benitez, M. A., & Lee, K. (2004, July 8). "Dedicated" Yeoh quits over Sars. *South China Morning Post*, p. A1.

Benitez, M. A., Lee, K., & Lo, E. (2004, July 9). Hospitals chief: We made no mistake. *South China Morning Post*, p. A1.

Chiu, W., & Galbraith, V. (2004). Calendar of events. In C. Loh & Civic Exchange (Eds.), *At the epicentre: Hong Kong and the SARS outbreak* (pp. xv–xxvii). Hong Kong: Hong Kong University Press.

Department of Health, Hong Kong Government. (2003, April 1). Protect yourself against atypical pneumonia. Available from http://www.info.gov.hk/dh.

Department of Health, Hong Kong Government. (2003, April 22). Prevent atypical pneumonia: For health to be bright/Get the hygiene right. Available from http://www.info.gov.hk/dh.

Department of Health by the Health, Welfare and Food Bureau, Hong Kong Government. (2003, April 22). SARS bulletin. Available from http://www.info.gov.hk/dh.

Department of Health, Hong Kong Government. (2003, April 25). A reminder for parents. Available from http://www.info.gov.hk/dh.

Department of Health, Hong Kong Government. (2003, April 7). Atypical pneumonia: Guidelines on inspection and disinfection of common parts of buildings. Available from http://www.info.gov.hk/dh.

Department of Health by the Department of Food and Environmental Hygiene, Hong Kong Government. (2003, April 9). Atypical pneumonia: Guidelines for employers and employees. Available from http://www.info.gov.hk/dh.

Department of Health, Hong Kong Government. (2003, March 20). Letter to doctors on atypical pneumonia outbreak in Hong Kong. Available from http://www.info.gov.hk/dh.

Department of Health, Hong Kong Government. (2003, March 24). Prevention of atypical pneumonia. Available from http://www.info.gov.hk/dh.

Department of Health, Hong Kong Government. (2003, March 26). Information for visitors to Hong Kong. Available from http://www.info.gov.hk/dh.

Department of Health, Hong Kong Government. (2003, March 27). Amendment to the quarantine and prevention of disease. Available from http://www.info.gov.hk/dh.

Department of Health, Hong Kong Government. (2003, March 29). Household cleaning day. Available from http://www.info.gov.hk/dh.

Department of Health, Hong Kong Government. (2003, March 31). Press release on isolation order. Available from http://www.info.gov.hk/dh.

Department of Health, Hong Kong Government. (2003, May 11). Daily AP bulletin for schools. Available from http://www.info.gov.hk/dh.

Department of Health, Hong Kong Government. (2003, May 11). Latest figures on severe acute respiratory syndrome. Available from http://www.info.gov.hk/dh.

Department of Health, Hong Kong Government. (2003, May 11). Travel advisory on atypical pneumonia. Available from http://www.info.gov.hk/dh.

Department of Health, Hong Kong Government. (2003, May 2). A summary of Hong Kong's hygiene laws. Available from http://www.info.gov.hk/dh.

Department of Social Welfare, Hong Kong Government. (2003, March 31). Emergency financial assistance for people affected by SARS. Available from http://www.info.gov.hk.

Hong Kong Government. (2003, March 31). Press release on transcript of Secretary's statement. Available from http://www.info.gov.hk.

Legislative Council Select Committee. (2004, July 7). *The handling of the Severe Acute Respiratory Syndrome outbreak by the government and the Hospital Authority.* Hong Kong: Hong Kong SAR Government.

Moy, P. (2004, April 21). Health Chief defends remarks. *South China Morning Post,* p. A4.

Sampathkumar, P., Temesgen, Z., Smith, T. F., & Thompson, R. L. (2003). SARS: Epidemiology, clinical presentation, management, and infection control measures. *Mayo Clinic Proceedings 78*, 882–890.

SARS Expert Committee. (2003a, October 2). *SARS in Hong Kong: From experience to action.* Hong Kong: Hong Kong SAR Government.

SARS Expert Committee. (2003b, October 2). *SARS in Hong Kong: From experience to action. A summary report of the SARS Expert Committee.* Hong Kong: Hong Kong SAR Government.

Wong, M. (2004, August 27). Hospital Authority director bows out. *South China Morning Post,* p. C4.

Wu, E. (2004, August 25). The cure that came at a cost. *South China Morning Post,* p. A16.

CHAPTER 4

Internet press freedom and online crisis reporting

The role of news Web sites in the SARS epidemic

Alice Y. L. Lee
Hong Kong Baptist University

This chapter examines the role played by news Web sites during the SARS crisis in two regions that have different degrees of Internet press freedom. Six online news sites in Hong Kong and mainland China were selected for investigation. The findings indicate that the news sites in Hong Kong, which enjoy a high degree of Internet press freedom, acted as "interactive crisis managers" and contributed in a number of ways to the management of the SARS crisis in the community. On the contrary, the news sites in mainland China, which are restricted by media censorship, served as the government's "online agent of containment." The findings also show that the news sites in both regions were able to offer efficient warnings, timely education, and a network of support during the crisis because of the unique characteristics of the Internet medium. However, due to the constraints on Internet press freedom, the Chinese sites were unable to take full advantage of the Internet medium to play a positive role in the management of the crisis.

This chapter examines the role played during the SARS crisis by news Web sites in two regions with different degrees of Internet press freedom – Hong Kong and mainland China. During the epidemic, 5,327 people in mainland China contracted the virus and 349 died, and in Hong Kong the cumulative number of SARS cases was 1,755 and the number of deaths was 299 (WHO 2003). Mainland China and Hong Kong had many similarities regarding the case of SARS. Both were "hot zones" of the epidemic, and both communities were thrown into a crisis situation after the initial outbreak. The online news media are well developed in both of these regions, and are already regarded as major news sources along with television and newspapers. Both are Chinese communities and they are geographically close.

In spite of these similarities, the two places do not have the same media system. The one in mainland China is a socialist press system while the one in Hong Kong is a free press system. Accordingly, they do not enjoy the same level of press freedom, and their online news media played very different roles during the SARS crisis. Previous studies of crisis reporting seldom touch on the issue of press freedom, as the free flow of information is taken for granted in Western societies, in which most of the studies were conducted. Moreover, research on the online news coverage of catastrophes is also scarce. Because the SARS crisis was widely covered by the online news media, and involves regions with different levels of press freedom, it offers a good opportunity to explore the relationship between Internet press freedom and online crisis reporting. Accordingly, it is theoretically and practically important to compare websites in Hong Kong and Mainland China in order to examine how the difference in Internet press freedom led to different ways of handling the crisis. (For a broader regional discussion of Internet press activities during the SARS crisis, see Lee 2005).

News Web sites and crisis reporting

The news media generally cover only those disasters or health crises that are regarded as newsworthy. The SARS epidemic was considered to be newsworthy because it met the industry criteria of the "assumed audience interest" principle (Singer & Endreny 1993) and the need to serve the community in a crisis. The epidemic fit the "newness" criterion because the SARS virus was a mysterious agent that caused a high number of fatalities. The epidemic was dramatic because the disease was lethal, and because it was totally unexplained. It came close to many people's doorstep because of its rapid spread through personal contact and air travel. Finally, the epidemic was not only a health crisis, but also an economic and political catastrophe in the areas that were worst affected. Apparently, the SARS epidemic met the media's "Ebola Standard" (Moeller 1999) of prominence, novelty, controversy, emotional appeal (terror), significance, and proximity.

The media in the areas most affected by SARS had an important role to play in the crisis. The literature of disaster reporting shows that the mass media play an essential role in warning citizens about natural threats, technological failures and health hazards. In an emergency situation, people need to obtain information from the mass media, both in terms of official warnings and unofficial news. More importantly, the way in which the mass media construct their reports about a catastrophe often determines how a society reacts toward the incident (Fischer 1998; Singer & Endreny 1993).

In recent years, comprehensive emergency management (CEM) has emerged as a professional and scientific means of responding to disasters. Through research and analysis, the elements that constitute effective management strategies that cut across specific incidents and disasters have been identified (Perry 1985). CEM is concerned with four phases of disaster management: mitigation, preparedness, response, and recovery (National Governors Association 1979). The most crucial contribution of the media is in the response phase, during which the media can help to save lives and avoid damage to property (Burkhart 1991). The media can guide the community to respond to a crisis by efficiently disseminating hazard information, warnings, and preparedness information. They can also help to control rumors, moderate panic, educate the public, and facilitate social relations. Therefore, the crisis management role of the mass media in the response stage can generally be grouped into five components: (a) delivering urgent information, (b) interpreting information arising from the crisis, (c) monitoring the authorities managing the crisis, (d) educating the public on issues related to the crisis, and (e) helping to construct care and support networks that aid the people affected by the crisis.

From the perspective of media theories, it is clear that the online news media have several unique characteristics that enable them to perform well in carrying out their social duties in a crisis.

As seen in Table 1, news sites can be accessed anywhere computers are available, and thereby reach an audience across regions and national borders. Online news is an immediate medium. The breaking news sections of online news sites have become instant sources of information during many recent disasters (Zollman 1997).

News sites also have an almost unlimited amount of space, and during a crisis are able to deliver a large amount of news and warnings to meet the rapidly changing information needs of a community that is suffering from physical dislocation and emotional strain. During epidemics such as SARS, news sites can easily set up data archives so that useful material can be accessed around the clock. By using the search function of news sites, community members can obtain educational information and understand how to take precautionary measures. The interactivity graphics and the multi-media function can facilitate the live demonstration of the correct ways of conducting precautionary activities. The interactive online message boards encourage suggestions and comments on handling a disaster, thereby providing certain monitoring on the crisis managers. Another valuable aspect of the personal nature of the Internet is its capacity for community building. During a disaster, there is a human impulse to reach out to others, and the Internet is capable of bridging the distance that often separates people by providing bulletin

Table 1. Characteristics of the online news media and crisis reporting functions

Crisis reporting function	Characteristics of the medium that particularly facilitate certain functions
Information dissemination and warnings	Online mass delivery
	Immediacy
	Data archive
	Unlimited space
	Active searching
Public education	Online mass delivery
	Immediacy
	Data archive
	Unlimited space
	Active searching
	Interactivity
	Multi-media function
Crisis interpretation and government monitoring	Interactivity
	Unlimited space
	Global access
Community building	Interactivity
	Connectivity
	Unlimited space
	Active searching
	Online access

boards and news chatrooms that enable people to communicate with one another and share their emotional reactions (Goldsborough 2001).

Internet press freedom and crisis reporting

According to Freedom House (Sussman 2000), the explosion of news and information on the World Wide Web in recent years has tempted many governments to consider placing restrictions on Internet content. The restriction of the free flow of news on the Internet infringes the fundamental right of free access to information, and attention has therefore been drawn to press freedom on the Internet. The Coordinating Committee of Press Freedom Organizations (2002) issued the following statement stressing the importance of preserving and extending press freedom on the Internet:

> News media in cyberspace and via international satellite broadcast should be afforded the same freedom of expression rights as traditional news media. Any text adopted by the World Summit of the Information Society should affirm this. A

free press means a free people. Press freedom on the Internet must be a fundamental characteristic of this and of any new communication system.

To ensure press freedom in cyberspace, a conference on "Press Freedom on the
Internet" was held in June 2003 (World Press Freedom Committee 2003a). Concerns were raised about the fact that "threats to Internet news have been apparent
in authoritarian societies such as China, Cuba and Iran since the dawn of the
Internet age itself" (Greene 2003, p. i). Chinese officials frequently attempt to
legitimize *Chinanet*, the Internet Service Provider system that acts as an intranet
instead of an Internet inside China, and thus prevents "undesirable" exchanges
with the outside world (Koven 2004). In China, huge amounts of financial and
human resources have been devoted to develop a secret "Golden Shield" program
that employs a cyber police force of some 30,000 persons to monitor the Internet
and identify "problematic" Internet users by the Ministry of Public Security and
the Ministry of Information Industry (He 2004). Scholars of Chinese studies have
often criticized the Chinese government for their censorship of Internet content
on political grounds, and for violating the principle of free flow of information
(Harwit & Clark 2001; Lacharite 2002).

   China has a poor record of press freedom. According to various surveys,
China's rating has remained at 80 and its press status is described as "not free"
(Sussman & Karlekar 2002; Karlekar 2003; Karlekar 2004). According to Freedom House, countries scoring 0–30 are regarded as having free media; 31–60 as
having partly free media; and 61–100 as having not free media. The 2004 press
freedom country report on China asserts that "the government promotes use of
the Internet, which it believes to be critical to China's economic development,
but regulates access, monitors use, and restricts and regulates content" (Karlekar
2004, p. 79). The findings of the Freedom on the Internet survey show that the
rating of China is "most restricted" whereas that of Hong Kong is listed as "least
restricted" (World Press Freedom Committee 2003b). Although Hong Kong was
handed back to China in 1997 and now operates under the "one country, two
systems" model, its traditionally free press is regarded as "relatively outspoken"
(Karlekar 2004, p. 79).

   Internet press freedom in fact is closely related to crisis reporting. The literature of crisis communication ranks "moving fast" as being the most important
principle for crisis management. Another important guideline is not to lie, because making a situation clear and transparent can reduce anxiety (Berge 1990;
Irvine & Millar 1998). In a crisis, the media need to provide accurate and timely
information to the affected members of society, and press freedom is therefore
crucial to the process of delivering emergency information. Crisis studies indicate
that information transparency in the press is essential to the successful execution

of a number of crisis management measures, such as alerting the people who are affected, easing social anxiety, mobilizing community resources, and boosting the morale of the rescuers and victims (Zhong 2003). Media observers clearly state that a free media is vital both in the fight against threatening diseases and in keeping the authorities honest (Chiu, Galbraith, & Loh 2004). Press freedom on the Internet is an important determinant of online disaster coverage and the stimulation of community response.

Internet news has flourished both in China and Hong Kong in the new millennium. At the end of June 2003, there were roughly 68 million Internet users in China, and the country now has the largest number of inhabitants online after the United States (AFP 2003a). Most of its online users use the Internet to seek news information (China Internet Network Information Center 2003). In Hong Kong, Internet use has also become popular and home audiences with access to news websites increased significantly in 2003. According to a Nielsen/NetRatings report, the traffic on news Web sites surged in Hong Kong as the war in Iraq began and SARS took hold. Half (50.3%) of all Internet users in Hong Kong visited a news or current affairs website during March 2003, compared with only 42% the year before. It has been reported that at the height of the SARS crisis in April 2003, the number of active Internet users increased by 13% over the previous month (Steyn 2003).

Research method

Because online users in China and Hong Kong both turned to the Internet for information about SARS during the epidemic, this study examines how the news Web sites in these two regions served their online readers during the crisis.Six news sites were selected for investigation from Hong Kong and mainland China. They include three from Hong Kong [*RTHK on the Internet* (Radio Television Hong Kong), *881903.com* (Commercial Radio), and *mingpao.com*], and three from mainland China [*cctv.com, eastday.com* and *dayoo.com*] (see Table 2). Content analysis was the major method of data analysis. There were two rounds of content analysis, the first comprising a quantitative analysis and the second a frame analysis.

March 31, 2003, was selected as the sample day for quantitative coding because this was when the Hong Kong government ordered the residents of the Amoy Gardens apartment complex to quarantine themselves at home following the announcement that 185 people who lived there had fallen ill with the virus (CNN 2003). The incident signaled to the world that the SARS outbreak was no longer contained within hospitals, but had spread to the community. A cross-sectional analysis of all of the six news sites was carried out. Although the quan-

Table 2. Online news coverage of the SARS crisis in sampled news sites on March 31, 2003

Region	Sampled sites	News coverage	
Hong Kong	www.rthk.org.hk	10.8% (121)	96.2% (1,082)
	www.881903.com	71.3% (802)	
	www.mingpao.com	14.1% (159)	
Mainland China	www.cctv.com.cn	1.7% (19)	3.8% (43)
	www.eastday.com	2.1% (24)	
	www.dayoo.com	0.0% (0)	
Total		100% (1,125)	100% (1,125)

titative data were drawn from only one day, a total of 1,125 online stories were recorded, including archive stories. The study covered all SARS related materials, including news stories, linked stories, and feature items in special reports. The news chain also included many news materials on SARS from before March 31. Using Krippendorff's (1980) alpha coefficient to test for inter-coder reliability, all variables have alpha higher than 0.7, which is the acceptable norm. The alpha coefficient for news theme is 0.809 while those for approach and source are 0.846 and 0.758 respectively.

The frame analysis looked at the ideological packages of the online media in Hong Kong and mainland China. The analysis draws on Gamson's (1988) work on interpretive packages. In this study, it is hypothesized that the two regions with different rankings of Internet press freedom generated different media discourses on the SARS outbreak. The media discourses can be conceived as a set of interpretive packages that gave meaning to the SARS epidemic, and in terms of a crisis management tool, also led the respective communities to respond to the epidemic in a particular way. According to Gamson and Modigliani (1989), such a package has an internal structure, and at its core is a central organizing idea or frame that is used to make sense of an ongoing stream of events. Metaphors, catchphrases, depictions, moral appeals, visual images, and other symbolic devices are some of the tools used in such packages (Gamson 1989; Ungar 2000). In this study, catchphrases related to the epidemic in news headlines as well as in the text of the news stories were recorded for analysis. Metaphors such as "battles" or "warriors" were identified. Visual images in online photos were also analyzed. The period for frame analysis is March 12 to July 5, 2003. These dates were selected because on March 12, the World Health Organization (WHO) issued a global health alert following the spread of SARS to medical staff in Vietnam and Hong Kong, which signaled the beginning of the epidemic. On July 5, the WHO declared that the outbreaks of SARS around the world had been contained. Archive stories and special reports on SARS on the six news sites during this period were included for examination.

News sites in Hong Kong: Interactive crisis managers

From March to July 2003, Hong Kong was under direct threat from SARS. It was one of the "hot zones," and was listed by the WHO as an affected area. Unsurprisingly, the crisis received heavy coverage from online news sites in Hong Kong. As the Internet penetration rate in Hong Kong exceeds 50%, news sites are already the third major source of news for local people (Zhu 2004). In addition, news sites were particularly popular during the epidemic because Hong Kong residents cut back their outdoor activities and spent more time at home. The findings of a Nielsen/NetRatings survey in Hong Kong clearly show an ongoing increase in Internet usage during the critical months of the SARS crisis (Steyn 2003).

The Hong Kong media did not play an active role in alerting the public in the early stages of the SARS epidemic. The SARS outbreak was first detected in Foshan in Guangdong province in November 2002, and by February 2003 had already spread to Guangzhou. According to Hong Kong journalists, local media people were too confident of Hong Kong's status as a first-class international city to imagine that such an epidemic would spread there (Fung 2003). By the time they discovered that the disease had reached Hong Kong and started to report on it in early March, the situation was already serious.

Fortunately, Hong Kong enjoys a high degree of press freedom and the online news media had a free hand to cover the SARS epidemic. During the response stage of the crisis, they were not only able to objectively report the situation but also capable of taking up the social roles of managing the crisis by using their unique interactive medium tools. Their crisis management tasks included delivering urgent information, interpreting information arising from the crisis, monitoring the government's SARS policies, educating the public to take precautionary measures and helping to construct support networks for the SARS victims.

Efficiently delivering crisis information and warnings

Many SARS reports point out that the existence of a free press was a distinct advantage for Hong Kong during the SARS crisis (Chiu, Galbraith, & Loh 2004). Sydney Chung, dean of the Faculty of Medicine at the Chinese University of Hong Kong, praised the local media for keeping the public informed, monitoring official actions, and playing a vital role in helping to contain the virus.

By the sample date of March 31, there were 530 cases of SARS in Hong Kong, and 13 fatalities. On that day, the residents of Amoy Gardens were quarantined, and the severe situation led the local media to fully devote their resources to the reporting of SARS. A total of 1,082 SARS stories, which included archive stories

Table 3. Roles of the online news media in the early stage of the SARS outbreak by news theme

Role	Hong Kong	Mainland China
Information dissemination	56.3% (1,110)	62.3% (66)
Public education	12.7% (251)	15.1% (16)
Crisis interpretation and government monitoring	13.2% (260)	8.5% (9)
Community building	16.3% (350)	13.2% (14)
Others	1.5% (29)	0.9% (1)
Total	100% (1,971 news themes)	100% (106 news themes)

Chi-square = 0.213 (not significant)

in special reports, were recorded on the news sites in Hong Kong (see Table 2). Among the SARS stories, 1,971 news themes were identified and divided into five categories. These categories represent the major social roles carried out by the SARS coverage, which include information dissemination, public education, crisis interpretation and community building. From Table 3, it can be seen that delivering information about the epidemic and the posting warnings were the most important functions performed by the news sites. About 1,110 online news items belong to this category. The local media sought to gather and disseminate the information that the community needed to adequately prepare and protect itself from the impact. On the one hand, the information included the latest infection statistics, details of new fatal cases, treatment methods, warnings from the health department, and the government's control measures, and on the other, the news media outlined the socio-economic impact of SARS and the social reactions to the outbreak.

As online news is an immediate medium, the online media busied themselves with the delivery of breaking news. In Hong Kong, 76.5% of online stories fell into this category. May Chan (personal communication, May 26, 2003), the News Director of *Commercial Radio*, said that she set up a SARS special report on the radio's website, *881903.com*, immediately after the outbreak was reported in Hong Kong because many people in the wider community were concerned about the crisis. The delivery of news about SARS through the Internet was also beneficial for potential visitors and overseas Chinese to Hong Kong, as they could learn about whether they should travel to the region and how they could take care of their relatives, friends, and property in Hong Kong. In fact, by March 31, all of the Hong Kong news sites had already packaged special reports to organize the material on SARS.

Another example of the usefulness of these features of news sites in handling the SARS crisis was the posting of the names of schools which announced their own closure before the education authority took any decisive action. In mid-March, the SARS epidemic had already spread in the community but the Hong Kong government still hesitated to close the schools. Some schools decided to take their own action and closed down in order to protect their students. The news websites, such as *mingpao.com*, were helpful by posting the announcements immediately on their education section so that students and parents could check the most updated school information on the Web round the clock. In the later stage, news sites also helped to post the names of the buildings that were affected by SARS so that citizens could check whether their neighborhood was safe. The building list was constantly updated, and the news sites became the places to understand how the disease spread geographically in the city.

Effectively educating the public

Because SARS was a new and highly contagious disease, it was very important to educate citizens about how to protect themselves. The online news media were very helpful in this respect because they were able to post a large quantity of educational materials about SARS for the reference of citizens. Table 3 indicates that by March 31, a total of 251 items on SARS-related educational themes could be found on the Hong Kong news sites. These news stories taught citizens about the nature of SARS, effective treatment for the virus, and how to protect themselves and seek assistance. Moreover, citizens were able to access these materials round the clock. For example, news sites used multi-media formats such as graphics, photos, and slides to show the proper way of putting on a facemask. The interactive function of the sites also allowed worried citizens to ask questions and seek advice from medical and nutrition specialists. Online readers could also download Chinese medicine prescriptions for strengthening their immune system to fight SARS.

Interpreting SARS and monitoring the government

Due to the high level of press freedom in Hong Kong, the online news media are able to monitor the government and challenge official views. Table 3 shows that 260 stories belong to the category of *analysis of the epidemic and commentary on policy*. The Hong Kong media challenged the government on a number of important issues, thereby pushing top officials to make quick decisions on a number of issues, such as determining whether SARS had broken out into the community in early March, whether the health authority should therefore alert citizens, whether schools should be closed to prevent the spread of the disease, whether the residents of Amoy Gardens should be sent to a quarantine camp, whether the government should release information on the buildings that were affected by SARS, and how the health authority could better protect frontline medical workers from contracting the disease.

Although phone-in radio programs did the best job of challenging official statements about the crisis, the online news media were also able to contribute through their interactive and connective functions by linking the reporting of these controversial issues with their chat rooms and message boards. The online forums were ideal places for citizens to join in the discussion, express their views, and question the government. For example, the forum of *mingpao.com* raised the question of "the medical professional collectively become SARS victims, what is your view?" The online news readers enthusiastically responded by urging the government to provide more protection to the medics. Other hot online discussion issues included how to properly treat the quarantined Amoy Gardens residents and how to take precautionary measures against further spreading of the disease. A senior multi-media editor of *mingpao.com* (Tsui, personal communication, June 19, 2003) pointed out that the SARS forum generated the highest input in the history of the *mingpao.com* site.

Forging a strong bond in the community

One of the greatest contributions of the Hong Kong online media to the management of the SARS crisis was community building. On the one hand, the media became a platform for social communication, and on the other, they adopted an advocacy role and became "campaign facilitators" in the fight against SARS (Chiu, Galbraith, & Loh 2004). Compared with the traditional media, the online news media played a unique role in providing social links between citizens. About 16% of online news themes on March 31 in Hong Kong were about community communication and sharing (see Table 3). Stories included government appeals, travel warnings, public announcements, community support, voluntary work, examples of heroism, the accounts of victims, and recovery stories. Through the news sites, citizens could get in touch with one another through sharing on the chatrooms and message boards. For example, online readers of *mingpao.com* could send their condolences and support to the quarantined Amoy Gardens residents in the camps.

The news sites were also effective in making the support of citizens known to the medical workers. *RTHK on the Internet* designed a special e-card and encouraged readers to send their support and appreciation to nurses and doctors in the hospitals. *Mingpao.com* also set up a section for posting their online readers' notes of thanks to the medics. The notes were also published in the print version of *Ming Pao Daily News*. A "One Person, One Facemask" campaign was launched by *Commercial Radio* through its website, *881903.com*, and its phone-in program, to raise funds to buy N95 masks for hospital workers who did not have access to such masks because the health authority did not supply enough. These campaigns helped to boost the morale of the frontline medical staff. Professor Joseph Sung Jao Yui, the Chief of the Department of Medicine and Therapeutics in the Prince of Wales Hospital, acknowledged that the citizens' support gave him and his colleagues a lot of encouragement (Sung 2004). Moreover, *RTHK on the Internet* listed a volunteer schedule to assist Hong Kong people to help each other during the crisis. In the later stage of the epidemic, *Mingpao.com* also launched a fundraising campaign to help children in the SARS victim families to continue their education.

Fighting back against SARS

The frame analysis finds that the crisis reporting of the Hong Kong online news media was characterized by an ideological package that was centered on "fighting the devastating virus." There are several sub-themes of this frame that promoted a "war" against the epidemic that was to be led by Hong Kong society. First, SARS was described as a fatal disease and citizens were regarded as vulnerable to its onslaught. The description of a "mysterious illness" projected uncertainty onto the unknown disease. The word *epidemic* was used all the time but not in a sensational sense.

However, the second sub-theme of "self-reliance" stressed that the medical system was not coping well with the outbreak, and that the government was not efficient in getting matters under control. Therefore, citizens had to protect themselves from the disease, and community members had to support each other, particularly in offering "weapons" to the frontline medical "warriors." This underlines the role of the media as crisis manager for the community. Both *mingpao.com* and *881903.com* assisted in promoting the SARS fund raising projects. The third subtheme of "fighting back against SARS" underscores the importance of the online media in co-opting the whole city into the campaign to fight against SARS. For example, *RTHK On the Internet* promoted the "We Shall Overcome" campaign on the Web and also posted volunteers' information. *Mingpao.com* posted a series of news stories featuring the brave stories of the SARS patients and their family members.

The fight against SARS in Hong Kong was, in fact, not seen as being led by the government but by social organizations, including the mass media. When SARS broke out, Hong Kong people accused the government of being slow and weak in its response. Since the government was seen as being so inefficient in handling the crisis, the media (including online news sites) collaborated with other social organizations to mobilize citizens to fight the "battle." This is evident in headline catchphrases such as "Heart links heart: The whole city is fighting against SARS," "Hong Kong is going to take off again!" and "Turning the adverse to miracle: The solidarity of Hong Kong people." Besides, metaphors like the "The self-reliance engineering project" of fighting SARS, the "war comrades" and "joining the combat" were frequently seen on news sites. Visually, both positive and negative images about SARS were objectively presented on the sites. There were numerous pictures of Amoy Gardens residents in quarantine camps. There were also pictures which showed how SARS victims overcame the mysterious disease. Overall, the visual images reflected what really happened in Hong Kong society.

Without any political constraints or censorship, the online news media in Hong Kong had a free reign in handling the crisis. They efficiently disseminated information to alert a large group of citizens. They were helpful in providing educational materials to prevent the disease from spreading, and the transparency of the information helped to control the rumors and reduce panic, both of which are crucial in crisis management. By framing the goal of crisis control as *a fight against SARS through self-reliance*, the online news media became a crisis coordinator and e-campaigner. They served as "interactive crisis managers."

China news sites: Online agent of containment

The foreign press described the SARS epidemic as "China's Chernobyl," which signifies both the seriousness of the incident and the secrecy that surrounded it. SARS was reported to have originated in Guangdong Province in November 2002. Although medical professionals filed a report to the health authority, the news was not released to the public and the press was constrained not to report it. In China, the press, which includes the Xinhua News Agency, cannot release any information without the approval of the government. It is only safe to report on official press conferences and speeches of the government leaders. There are also regulations controlling the postings on web sites. If the postings are considered to have a bad influence on social stability, then the sites cannot post them (AFP 2003a).

In the case of SARS, the news media in China were unable to assist the public just when they were most needed. Despite the crisis, the media were silenced on the issue of SARS. This study finds that in the early stages, only a small number of stories on SARS could be found on China's online news sites. April 17, 2003, was the turning point of the media blackout. As a result of international pressure, the Politburo ordered wider reporting about SARS. On April 20, 2003, the Health Minister, Zhang Wenkang, and the Mayor of Beijing, Meng Xuenong, were removed from their positions for covering up the spread of SARS (BBCi 2003; Zhang & Benoit, in press) and the first press conference on SARS was conducted by the News Office of the State Department. The green light was then given for covering the crisis. However, the media, including news sites, still did not have a free hand in reporting the crisis. They had to follow the state's instructions and became the government's "agent of containment."

From information blockade to information overflow

On the sample day of March 31, 2003, only 43 SARS-related stories, which include archive stories, were found on the sampled news sites in China (see Table 2). Compared with the 1,082 stories in Hong Kong, China's coverage was minimal. There were 19 stories on *cctv.com*, 24 stories on *eastday.com*, and no SARS stories at all on *dayoo.com*. *Dayoo.com* is a Guangzhou-based news site, and at that time press censorship was particularly tight in Guangdong province, the capital of which is Guangzhou.

Usually, news sites in China offer a large amount of up to the minute breaking news. However, on March 31, there was neither breaking news nor any special coverage of SARS. Among the 43 stories about SARS found on the sites, most presented an optimistic view of the outbreak. This may be due to the fact that 76.2% of the news stories depended on government sources and 72.1% of the stories came from the official news agencies. More importantly, only a quarter of the coverage was about the SARS situation in mainland China itself, with the rest being about the epidemic in Hong Kong and Taiwan. These "outside" stories were put in the "Hong Kong, Macao and Taiwan News" section. Apparently, the online news media in China hesitated to report on the crisis on the mainland, and were not able to alert the public about the lethal virus. At that time, online journalists understood that they were under the surveillance of the internal cyber security unit to make sure that they did not leak what were deemed to be state secrets.

By March, SARS had already spread to many provinces in China, including Beijing. The media cover-up in the early stage of the epidemic meant that China had lost the chance to stop the disease from spreading to other provinces and the rest of the world. Instead of controlling the rumors and reducing panic, the media blackout stimulated the dissemination of rumors through text messaging, and generated a countrywide panic (Du 2003; Xu & Yan 2003).

However, by mid-April, after Chinese leaders Wen Jiabao and Hu Jintao announced that there should be no cover-up of the epidemic, the online news media began to organize special SARS packages, and online news sites were flooded with material about SARS. For example, the Guangdong sample site, *dayoo.com*, switched from complete silence about SARS to actively reporting developments in the crisis. A special report package entitled "Eliminate SARS and Say No to the Epidemic" was created, and a wide variety of information about SARS was included in the package. The news sites *cctv.com* and *eastday.com* also developed special report packages, which included nationwide outbreak updates, government control measures, advice from experts, medical research on SARS, and inquiry hotlines. The amount of SARS coverage online was astonishing, both in terms of quantity and comprehensiveness.

This impressive coverage was an effort to follow the government instruction to better inform the public about the disease. The online media were regarded as being particularly suitable to carry out this role of information deliverer because they are fast, mass-oriented, have no space limit, are able to cross provincial boundaries, are interactive, and have diverse news presentation formats (Dong 2003).

The SARS epidemic was particularly serious in big cities like Guangzhou and Beijing, and the Internet penetration rates in both cities are very high. People in the search-engine business reported that surfing for SARS data was popular among China's Internet users. Baidu, a Chinese-language search engine based in Beijing and SinoLinx, the news section of the *Xianzai.com* Web information service for foreigners in China, announced that SARS was their number one search string during the epidemic. With people staying indoors to avoid SARS, the Internet and text messages were the first to inform the wired population about SARS and the efforts that were being taken to control it, and Web sites had a higher hit rate than normal (Jen-siu 2003). Although people in China did not fully believe what the sites reported, the online media were a convenient way to check public announcements and government policy on SARS.

From misleading to educating

Table 3 shows that by March 31, only 16 items on SARS-related educational themes were found on the Chinese news sites, compared with the 251 items that were found on the Hong Kong sites. Compared with their Hong Kong counterparts, the online news media failed completely to educate the Chinese people about this mysterious disease. Rumors spread in southern China that vinegar was effective against the virus, and subsequently many people rushed out to buy vinegar products. Instead of helping people to take precautions against the virus, misinformation stirred social instability, and many workers from other provinces left the big cities in fear, which served to spread the virus even wider and faster.

However, after April 2003, the government and the health authority made full use of the Internet to disseminate timely public health education about the epidemic. The online news media launched a massive propaganda campaign on the Web to tell their readers about SARS and ways in which it could be avoided. The targets of the education campaign were not only ordinary community members, but also medical professionals. Initially, medical staff knew little about the preventive measures against the virus, and had to rely on information they found on Web sites (Ma 2003). The health authority even uploaded training VCDs for doctors to online news sites (Dong 2003).

From neglecting the people to consolidating the community

During the epidemic, the *Financial Times* (2003) described China as "a country that does not take care of its people." The SARS cover-up clearly illustrated that Chinese officials put national reputation and economic development before the lives of the population. However, after the change in official policy, the online media became tools of propaganda, and called upon the whole nation to stand together to fight the disease. The metaphor of "people's war" was frequently articulated in the crisis coverage. It was like the old-styled campaign (*yundong*) aiming at uniting the will of the masses, all social institutions and political organizations into a "fortress" (He 2004). This study finds that the online news sites were able to post many exclusive articles on SARS victims and medical workers, and featured stories about them carrying out their duties and fighting the virus. The heroic deeds of the frontline medical staff, the concern of the national leaders, and the speeches of government officials in press conferences were delivered on the Web through multi-media devices, such as photos, slides, sound clips, and video clips. Although there was criticism that the reporting was too sensational, those stories were regarded as useful in consolidating the nation during the crisis (Cai 2003; Dong 2003).

From censorship to containment: Everything was under control

Without Internet freedom, the online news media in China had little involvement in monitoring the government. Even after the shift in official policy in April, the online news media were still under tight control, and dared not do anything that was not instructed by the government. The frame analysis reveals that the ideological content of the coverage in China was that of a "containment package."

The frame of containment was constructed around a number of themes. The first, which was "contagious but not horrible and incurable," comforted frightened people by denying that the virus was unbeatable, and the catchphrase, "early discovery, early diagnosis, early reporting, early quarantine and early treatment will lead to early recovery" was widely publicized throughout the nation (*Eastday.com* 2003). On *CCTV.com*, doctors were invited to answer online readers' questions and talk about precautionary measures. *Eastday.com* also set up special sections such as "Medical Professional's Recommendations," "Precaution Knowledge," and "Precaution Prescriptions" which included Chinese medicine prescriptions as well as psychological prescriptions. While the SARS crisis was often addressed as an "epidemic" in Hong Kong, it was hyped as "deadly illness," "killer disease," "mysterious disease" on the American and British news sites. However, in mainland China, SARS was neutrally named as "atypical pneumonia" and the word "outbreak" was seldom seen on their sites.

The second theme of "everything is under control" described the virus as being well contained and controlled, and the online reports highlighted that "the whole nation is whole-heartedly fighting SARS together." Online sites were flooded with visual images featuring the visits of top leaders to the medical professionals, the bravery of the frontline medics, and the smiling faces of recovering patients. The picture depicting Premier Wen Jiabao holding a SARS victim's baby at the Amoy Gardens in Hong Kong was widely posted on the mainland news sites. Online readers could often see the pictures of national leaders visiting various affected zones without putting their masks on. Moreover, as foreign media described Beijing as a "ghost town," the Chinese sites portrayed Beijing as the "battle field" where the war on SARS was fought and the victory was finally gained. The nurses and doctors were addressed as "white gown warriors" or "white gown angels," and they were reported as facing the SARS challenge with bravery.

Lastly, the containment package urged the Chinese people to be "scientific and modern." In the special reports section of many news sites, there were interviews on medical experts and psychologists, talking about how to use the scientific methods and attitudes to meet the challenge of SARS. A lot of space was also devoted to publishing research developments on SARS around the world. The visual images on the news sites always presented the nurses and doctors with masks, gloves and medical garb on, emphasizing their professional image. Besides, the endorsement of the bans on spitting and the eating of wild animals, and the promotion of the fighting of the epidemic with a scientific attitude underlay many SARS stories. Another catchphrase "eliminate SARS and say no to its prevalence" demonstrated the government's determination to bring SARS under control through a scientific battle.

One great feature of online news sites is their interactive forums and, as in Hong Kong, message boards and chatrooms in China were flooded with SARS-related messages during the later SARS period. For example, the forum on the online version of the *People's Daily* received more than 6,000 postings about SARS (Dong 2003). However, the online forums were heavily censored, and only those views that towed the official line could be posted (AFP 2003a). In our sampled sites, for example, postings that challenged the official views were rarely found. Most of the postings expressed the gratitude of readers for the bravery of the frontline medical staff, emphasized the importance of solidarity in fighting the epidemic, and offered positive suggestions for handling the crisis. According to the editors of these news sites, "negative" postings could result in fines or punishment. In fact, during the epidemic, there was even tighter control of the Internet. In April, a 17-year-old girl was arrested for posting "harmful information" in a central Chinese Internet chatroom (AFP 2003b).

Table 3 presents the quantitative data of the roles performed by news sites in both Hong Kong and China in the early stage of the outbreak. In the beginning of the SARS crisis, news media in these two regions both put emphasis on disseminating information. Chi-square test shows that there was no significant difference between the patterns on crisis reporting between sites in these two regions. However, while the patterns were the same, the volumes of the coverage differed greatly (see Table 2). The China sites only offered 43 stories in contrast with 1,082 stories provided by the Hong Kong sites. The online news media in both regions were supposed to take up the same crisis management roles of delivering urgent information, educating the public, interpreting the crisis and building a care network. However, due to the information control of the Chinese government, the mainland news sites failed to perform their duties in the early response stage of the SARS crisis.

In the later stage, the mainland news sites devoted huge resources and space in delivering SARS information and educating the general public. On the surface, it seems that they were doing the same as their Hong Kong counterparts. But frame analysis shows what the online sites had done was part of the government's containment scheme. Online crisis reporting in China was framed in a unique way. During the crisis, the Chinese central government set up a containment policy which included collecting facts, establishing a crisis management team, releasing selected information and framing the issue. The government officials aimed at "setting up a tone to inspire public emotion, reconstructing the image of the government as being capable of managing the crisis, and influencing public opinion so as to stabilize the society and maintain social order" (He 2004, p. 192). This study shows that the Hong Kong news sites were able to reflect the objective reality of the impact of SARS on the community and encouraged the build up of a self-reliant supporting network in the civic society. On the contrary, mainland news sites served the government's top-down SARS containment campaign (*yundong*) by providing selected information and one-sided public opinion. Chinese communication scholars pointed out that "an authoritarian system often creates asymmetric information system . . . which provides an opportunity for bureaucrats to lie without being noticed, and to 'sell' information for their material benefits" (He 2004, p. 182). The containment package of the mainland sites is obviously characterized by this asymmetric feature.

Freedom on the Internet and crisis reporting online

In disasters and catastrophes, the media are not only major partners of governments, but are also important members of the crisis management team in society. In the digital age, and with more and more people going online, news Websites will play an increasingly significant role in covering disasters and performing crisis management duties. There are comments that all governments (both authoritarian and democratic) tend to control information about an uncertain epidemic. The difference lies in the existence of a free press so that a government is under pressure to share information with its people (He 2004). Therefore, it is essential for the online news media to have a free hand to perform their duties. Internet press freedom is an important determinant to the news sites' crisis management performance.

In the case of SARS, the online news media, along with the traditional media, played a satisfactory role as an "interactive crisis manager" in Hong Kong. In terms of public education and community building, the interactive nature of the online medium enabled them to carry out these functions much better than their traditional counterparts. However, the online news media in mainland China were unable to take advantage of this new technology to alert and inform their readers. The discrepancy between the performance of the online news media in the two regions was due to the difference in Internet press freedom. The Chinese authorities were aware of the utility of online news sites, and made full use of them as propaganda tools to help contain the disease and maintain social stability in the later stages of the epidemic. They regarded the online news media as powerful "online foot soldiers" in the fight against SARS (Dong 2003), and this phenomenon relates to the old saying that technology itself is neutral, and its proper use depends on each society's socio-political and structural characteristics. In the later stage of the outbreak, the mainland online news media put a lot of efforts on crisis reporting but they did not win the trust of the Chinese people. Chinese people chose to depend on getting their SARS information through their

SMS channels. Moreover, the whole Chinese society was not unified to form a bottom-up care and supporting network. What the news sites in China could do was limited to serving as the government's "online agent of containment."

In sum, then, this study shows that Internet press freedom is certainly an important determinant in shaping the nature of online crisis reporting, and affects the role of the online media in crisis management. Sussman (2003) at Freedom House is pessimistic about the near future of press freedom on the Internet, and he predicts that the Internet will be subject to systemic and content controls by authoritarian rulers and even in some democracies. This study reveals that Internet censorship paralyzed the crisis management function of the online news media and further led to the loss of human life in mainland China during the SARS crisis. Therefore, safeguarding press freedom on the Internet is an urgent issue that must be addressed by today's high technology societies.

References

Agence France-Presse. (2003a, April 7). Mainland media gag is extended to the Internet. *South China Morning Post*, p. A3.

Agence France-Presse. (2003b, April 4). Mainland girl arrested over Web chatroom posting. *SCMP.com*. Retrieved April 9, 2003 from http://technology.scmp.com/techinternet/ZZZMTCV80ED.html.

BBCi. (2003, April 20). China faces up to virus threat. Asia Pacific section, *BBCi*. Retrieved June 9, 2003 from http://news.bbc.co.uk/2/hi/asia-pacific/2961819.stm.

Berge, D. T. (1990). *The first 24 hours: A comprehensive guide to successful crisis communications*. Oxford: Basil Blackwell.

Burkhart, F. N. (1991). *Media, emergency warnings, and citizen response*. Oxford: Westview Press.

Cai, W. (2003, May). Viewing news editorial policy from the SARS coverage. *International News*, pp.10–13.

China Internet Network Information Center. (2003). *12th statistical survey on Internet development in China*. Beijing: China Internet Network Information Center.

Chiu, W., Galbraith, V., & Loh, C. (2004). The media and SARS. In C. Loh & Civic Exchange (Eds.), *At the epicentre: Hong Kong and the SARS outbreak* (pp. 195–214). Hong Kong: Hong Kong University Press.

CNN. (2003). Timeline: SARS outbreak. Retrieved July 31, 2003, from http://edition.cnn.com/SPECIALS/2003/sars.

Coordinating Committee of Press Freedom Organizations. (2002). The statement of Vienna: press freedom on the Internet. Retrieved April 5, 2003 from www.wpfc.orgPress%20Freedom%20on%20the%20Internet%20Statement.htm.

Dong, M. J. (2003, July). Competing to be the online foot soldiers in SARS reporting: The powerful Peopledaily.com. *Journalism Frontline*, pp. 64–66.

Du, J. F. (2003). The changing rumors. *China Media Report*, 2(4), 95–102.

Eastday.com. (2003). Prevention of contracting SARS by applying scientific method. *Eastday. com*. Retrieved August 10, 2003, from http://sars.eastday.com.

Financial Times. (2003, April 8). A country that does not take care of its people. *Financial Times,* p. 19.

Fischer, H. W. III. (1998). *Response to disaster: Fact versus fiction and its perpetuation* (2nd ed.). New York: University Press of America.

Fung, T. H. (2003). *Cable TV and SARS reporting.* Paper presented at the Conference of Digital News, Social Change and Globalization Conference, December 11–12, Hong Kong.

Gamson, W. A. (1988). The 1987 distinguished lecture: A constructionist approach to mass media and public opinion. *Symbolic Interaction, 11*(2), 161–174.

Gamson, W. A. (1989). News as framing. *American Behavioral Scientist, 33*(2), 157–161.

Gamson, W. A., & Modigliani, A. (1989). Media discourse and public opinion on nuclear power: A constructionist approach. *American Journal of Sociology, 95*,1–37.

Goldsborough, R. (2001). In a crisis, old media trump new media. *Community College Week, 14*(7), 19.

Greene, M. (2003). Foreword. In World Press Freedom Committee (Ed.), *Press freedom on the Internet* (pp. i–iii). New York: Press Freedom on the Internet.

Harwit, E., & Clark, D. (2001). Shaping the Internet in China: Evolution of political control over network infrastructure and content. *Asian Survey, 4* (3), 377–408.

He, B (2004). SARS and freedom of the press: Has the Chinese government learnt a lesson? In J. Wong & Y. Zheng (Eds.), *The SARS epidemic: Challenges to China's crisis management* (pp. 181–198). London: World Scientific.

Irvine, R. B., & Millar, D. P. (1998). *Crisis management and communication: How to gain and maintain control.* San Francisco: IABC.

Jen-siu, M. (2003, May 20). Net used to spread news on virus. *South China Morning Post,* p. T7.

Karlekar, K. D. (Ed.). (2003). *Freedom of the press 2003: A global survey of media independence.* New York: Freedom House.

Karlekar, K. D. (Ed.). (2004). *Freedom of the press 2004: A global survey of media independence.* New York: Freedom House.

Koven, R. (2004). In defiance of common sense: The practical effects of international press restrictions. In K. D. Karlekar (Ed.), *Freedom of the press 2004: A global survey of media independence* (pp. 41–47). New York: Freedom House.

Krippendorff, K. (1980). *Content analysis: An introduction to its methodology.* Beverly Hills, CA: Sage.

Lacharite, J. (2002). Electronic decentralization in China: A critical analysis of Internet filtering policies in the People's Republic of China. *Australian Journal of Political Science, 37,* 333–346.

Lee, A. Y. L. (2005). Between global and local: The glocalization of online news coverage on the trans-regional crisis of SARS. *Asian Journal of Communication, 15,* 255–273.

Ma, J. (2003, May 24). Medics forge a strong bond in frontline battle. *South China Morning Post,* p. A4.

Moeller, S. D. (1999). *Compassion fatigue: How the media sell disease, famine, war and death.* New York: Routledge.

National Governors Association. (1979). *Emergency preparedness project: Final report.* Washington, DC: National Governors Association, Center for Policy Research.

Perry, R. W. (1985). *Comprehensive emergency management: Evacuating threatened populations.* Greenwich, CT: JAI Press.

Singer, E., & Endreny, P. M. (1993). *Reporting on risk: How the mass media portray accidents, diseases, disasters, and other hazards.* New York: Russell Sage Foundation.

Steyn, P. (2003). *SARS stimulates ongoing growth in Internet usage in Hong Kong.* Hong Kong: Nielsen/NetRatings.

Sung, J. Y. (2004). *Not the same sky.* Hong Kong: ET Press.

Sussman, L. R. (2000). Censor dot gov: The Internet and press freedom 2000. Freedom House: press freedom survey 2000. Retrieved April 5, 2003, from www.freedomhouse.org/pfs2000/sussman.html.

Sussman, L. R. (2003). Press freedom on the Internet at risk in the short term. In World Press Freedom Committee (Ed.), *Press freedom on the Internet* (pp. 21–28). New York: World Press Freedom Committee.

Sussman, L. R., & Karlekar, K. D. (Eds.). (2002). *The annual survey of press freedom 2002.* New York: Freedom House.

Ungar, S. (2000). Hot crisis and media reassurance: A comparison of emerging diseases and Ebola in Zaire. *British Journal of Sociology, 49*(1), 36–56.

World Health Organization. (2003, September 23). *Summary of probable SARS cases with onset of illness from 1 November 2002 to 31 July 2003.* Retrieved December 21, 2003 from http://www.who.int/csr/sars/country/table2003_09_23/en/.

World Press Freedom Committee. (2003a). The purpose of statement – Internet conference. Retrieved on April 5, 2003 from www.wpfc.org/internet-conference-links.htm.

World Press Freedom Committee. (2003b). Press freedom on the Internet: A groundbreaking conference examining issues of press freedom in the Internet age. New York: World Press Freedom Committee.

Xu, F. M., & Yan, S. J. (2003). The rumor communication in the Guangzhou SARS epidemic. *Journalism University, 78,* 36–43.

Zhang, E., & Benoit, W. (in press). Government image restoration or destruction: Former minister Zhang's Discourse on SARS. Cresskill, NY: Hampton Press.

Zhong, X. (2003, May). Crisis effect and media functions. *International News,* pp. 19–23.

Zhu, J. (2004). *Diffusion and use of the Internet in Hong Kong from 2000–2003.* Paper presented at the First APIRA Conference on "Information Statistics of the Internet: Measurement, Analysis and Applications." August 19–20, 2004, Hong Kong.

Zollman, P. M. (1997). Community disaster coverage. *Editor and Publisher, 130*(38), 34.

PART II

Constructions of SARS
on the Chinese Mainland

CHAPTER 5

Party journalism vs. market journalism

The coverage of SARS by *People's Daily* and *Beijing Youth News*

Huang Xiaoyan and Hao Xiaoming
Nanyang Technological University

This study examines how *People's Daily,* an organ of the Chinese Communist Party, and *Beijing Youth News,* a market-oriented newspaper, covered the SARS crisis in 2003. A qualitative analysis of the SARS-related stories shows that the two newspapers basically followed the Party's overall policy towards information management regarding the epidemic. The newspapers' censorship and publicity of information about the epidemic were based on the Party's strategies rather than their own editorial decisions. However, the two newspapers also had some important differences in handling news about the Party leaders, the medical workers and the public. While *People's Daily* tended to follow the Party line in its daily reports about the epidemic, *Beijing Youth News* was more likely to follow its bottom line by presenting stories of greater relevance to the public.

The research literature has described the Chinese press as an instrument of the Communist Party to propagate its political line and policies (Pan 2000). As such, the official press sees itself as the Party's "mouthpiece" and supports a "commandist system" (Lee 1990; Pan 2000). Despite China's economic and political reforms in recent decades, the Chinese Communist Party's fundamental concept of political communication and the propagandist role of media remain largely unchanged (Du 2004; Esarey 2006; Lee 2003; Zhao 1998).

No major disagreement has been aired regarding the fundamental nature of the Chinese press, but it cannot be denied that China's reforms have also brought some unprecedented changes to the Chinese media, at least in terms of their financial operations. The discarding of the planned economy resulted in the redistribution of wealth from the central government to local authorities, enterprises and individuals, making the government incapable of financing the press (Zhao 1998). In the meantime, the expanding market provided an ideal environment for the growth of China's advertising industry, which has become the most important source of revenue for the Chinese press.

The gradual severance of government subsidy to the news media since the 1980s has led to "the expansion of China's media marketplace in terms of number of outlets and variety of offerings" (Polumbaum 1994, p. 115). Major changes include the revival of the popular evening newspapers in the mid-1980s; the expansion of space and launching of weekend editions by existing newspapers in the early 1990s; and the rise of metropolitan newspapers in the mid-1990s (Huang 2001; Yu 1994; Zhao 1998). In general, these new publications are offshoots of major newspapers run directly by the Party and government, which have had to keep their official façade and are inflexible for the market. These new mass appeal papers, which emphasize breaking events and human interest stories, soon got the upper hand in the market.

"Commercialization has created some opportunities for relative autonomy where Party control and market imperatives intertwine" (Zhao 1998, p. 94), but to what extent the market-oriented newspapers differ from the mainstream Party and government newspapers when it comes to the basic functions of the press remains a question. These market-oriented newspapers have certainly helped to diversify news as they offer more space and are less pressured to report the "official" news. But does this mean that they serve as real alternatives to their parent newspapers when it comes to the coverage of China's major events and issues? The answer to such a question is of great significance because the market-oriented newspapers have already replaced the mainstream Party newspapers for a significant proportion of China's readers. If they construct a competing version of China's reality for their readers, those readers would naturally perceive the world differently from readers of the mainstream Party newspapers, which are designed to give the official version of reality to the Chinese public.

Among the realities that newspapers frequently help their readers interpret are natural disasters, which have often been purposely ignored by the Chinese press (Zhang 1997). Concerns about the risk of public panic and potential damage to the image of the Chinese leadership often make the authorities hesitant to publicize news about natural disasters. For example, during the four months after the first SARS case was diagnosed in China's Guangdong province in November 2002, the Chinese government imposed a virtual news blackout. As a result of this censorship, the epidemic found time to travel both inside and outside China, resulting in a total of 8,098 cases and 774 deaths worldwide by the end of July 2003 (World Health Organization 2003). The consequence could have been even worse had it not been for Dr. Jiang Yanyong, a retired army surgeon, whose exposure to the international media of the government's cover-up concerning the severity of the epidemic finally persuaded the Chinese government to publicize the problem.

The SARS epidemic was no doubt one of the more important crises faced by the Chinese Communist Party since the Cultural Revolution. At stake was not only public health but also the credibility of the Chinese Communist Party and government, which initially tried to cover up the spread of the epidemic. The SARS crisis therefore offers an ideal setting to compare the official and the market-oriented media. The results will not only offer guidelines for journalists and the public in handling future crises, but also allow us to see the impact of structural changes in the Chinese media system over the years.

Method

To explore the differences between the Party-oriented and market-oriented newspapers in their handling of major events and issues related to the SARS crisis, this study compares the news coverage of *People's Daily*, an organ of the Chinese Communist Party, with that provided by *Beijing Youth News,* a market-oriented newspaper run by the Communist Youth League of Beijing municipality.

Although both *People's Daily* and *Beijing Youth News* have to subject their content to the overall Party and state controls, they differ in terms of their relative allegiance to the Communist Party and the market. Being an organ of the Communist Party, *People's Daily* is closely watched by Party propagandists whose job is to make sure that the newspaper reflects the official Party line. It is read by Communist Party officials for directives from the central authorities of the Communist Party. *Beijing Youth News,* on the other hand, has evolved into a commercial newspaper over the years. Despite its ownership by the Beijing Communist Youth League, *Beijing Youth News* is meant for the common folks, whose taste dictates the paper's editorial content. The contrast between the two newspapers reflects different orientations in China's newspaper operations today – Party journalism vs. market journalism. A comparison of the two newspapers in their coverage of SARS allows us to see whether loyalty to the Party and loyalty to the market have indeed resulted into a difference between the two newspapers in terms of helping the nation to overcome the SARS crisis.

The time frame for this study begins on February 11, 2003, when the government of Guangdong Province announced the outbreak of SARS in the province, and ends on June 4, 2003, when China recorded no new SARS cases and no new SARS-related deaths for the first time. All stories related to SARS published during this period by *People's Daily* and *Beijing Youth News* were obtained from their websites, yielding a total of 1,317 stories from *People's Daily* and 1,591 from the *Beijing Youth News*.

Because the two newspapers differ in editorial space and reporting style, we took a qualitative approach to comparing their coverage. We examined their respective presentations of the epidemic through a comparison of their reports day by day to discover the extent to which they differed in terms of a number of factors. We first examined the accuracy of the news reports by checking if there were contradictory reports later and if they differed from information obtained from WHO and other sources. Then we examined the timeliness of the reports by checking how fast the outbreak of the epidemic and various stages of its development were reported. Other factors examined included context, comprehensiveness, sources, diversity of coverage, human interest, reporting style, and so forth. We tried to read the news as ordinary readers would have in order to see if we could get different perceptions of the epidemic by reading the two newspapers.

Although this study follows the general approach of framing analysis (Goffman 1974) with the understanding that news frame organizes everyday reality (Tuchman 1978), it did not analyze the news discourse by examining the usual framing devices such as syntactical structure, script structure, thematic structure, and rhetorical structure (Pan & Kisichi 1993). Instead, it focused on the major players in the news. At its heart, news is about people and what they do. This is even truer for the coverage of SARS, which would not have caught so much media attention if not for the fact that it victimized thousands and affected millions of people. In that sense, news about SARS is really news about people rather than the disease itself. Therefore, we focused our analysis on the main characters in the news.

Our initial reading of the SARS stories identified three groups of people as major players in SARS-related news. The first group consists of Party and government leaders, who are always prominently covered by the Chinese media due to their propaganda role. The second group is composed of the health workers, including the medical scientists, doctors and nurses, who played a major role in handling the crisis. The last group is the general public, who are not only readers of the news but also potential victims of the epidemic.

By focusing on these three groups, we aimed to accomplish three objectives. First, we attempted to identify the major sources of information. New sources play an important role in framing the news and molding readers' perception. The selection of sources is determined not only by their knowledge of and closeness to the news event, but also by their prominence and authoritativeness, as well as journalistic bias of the reporters and editors. Second, we wanted to see whose opinions and interpretations dominated the news. In typical Chinese journalism, news aims for consensus rather than diversity of opinion. The real test for the loyalty of the Chinese media happens when their two masters, the Party and state on one hand and the public as consumers on the other, differ in their concerns and views about the issues involved. By examining the dominant views expressed through the news, we would be able to see if the market-oriented *Beijing Youth News* really differed from the Party-oriented *People's Daily*. Lastly, we aimed to see whose activities made up the news. Did the news center on the activities of leaders, the health workers or the general public? Different approaches may reflect the importance the media attach to the different groups as well as journalists' understanding of the news. Again, this would allow us to see if the two newspapers might have taken different approaches to SARS coverage in line with the differences in the primary objective of their news production.

Coverage of the disease

Both newspapers' coverage of the development of the epidemic is in line with the Party's stance in handling the disease. Before April 20, neither *People's Daily* nor *Beijing Youth News* provided accurate statistics on the outbreak and spread of the epidemic. Though the first cases of SARS in Guangdong province were diagnosed in November 2002, neither newspapers published any stories on the disease before the Guangdong Health Bureau made a public announcement about it on February 11, 2003, on which day the two newspapers only carried a brief report. When the first SARS case occurred in Beijing on March 1, 2003, neither newspaper reported the case.

The coverage of the spread of the disease was crafted in such a way that even the WHO's global alert warning, the inclusion of Beijing on its list of SARS affected areas, and its advice against traveling to Hong Kong and Guangdong were ignored by both newspapers. On March 27, when the WHO put Beijing on its list of SARS affected areas, *Beijing Youth News* carried its second SARS-related story on its second page, reporting only two suspected cases and eight confirmed cases in the capital. Four days later, however, it published on its ninth page an unusual story headlined "Gauze Masks out of Stock for Several Days," which indirectly addressed the issue of SARS. On the other hand, *People's Daily* had no follow-up stories on SARS until April 3, when both papers broke the silence by reporting the April 2 meeting of the State Council on the SARS issue as well as an interview with Health Minister Zhang Wenkang, who claimed "it is safe to live, work and travel in China." To support the Minister's claim, both newspapers carried stories on how foreign tourists felt it was safe to be in Beijing.

In their later reports, both papers focused on offering tips on how to prevent the disease and gave more space to stories about the recovered patients than to stories about those suffering from the disease. On April 8, both papers claimed that the incidence of the epidemic was dropping in Beijing. In the ensuing days, both papers carried a series of stories on recovered SARS patients in Beijing and elsewhere. Not a single report on the international criticism of China's secretive handling of the SARS epidemic could be found in either newspaper. Instead, both papers primed the news to show how accurate the government-released figures were.

After April 3, SARS-related news became an indispensable part of the front page of *Beijing Youth News. People's Daily,* on the other hand, carried most SARS related news on inside pages. Only stories like "Chinese Government Has the Ability to Control SARS" were able to grace its front page. Compared with *Beijing Youth News, People's Daily* also seemed to have gone further in priming the news more favorably toward the government. When a WHO team met the Mayor of Beijing on April 15, *People's Daily* gave the headline "WHO Experts Extremely Impressed by Beijing's Innovative Measures to Control SARS," while *Beijing Youth News* chose to say that "International Cooperation Is Needed to Control SARS." Neither paper reported the WHO team's criticism of the Chinese government for vastly underreporting the epidemic outbreak in China.

Both papers chose to downplay the role played by Dr. Jiang Yanyong, whose exposure of the cover-up of the SARS situation by the Chinese government led to the Chinese government's about-face. Neither newspaper chose to report the doctor's letter to the media. However, Dr. Jiang's name did appear once in a *Beijing Youth News* column in which he was briefly quoted as saying that "doctors should tell the truth, otherwise, more people will lose their lives and our nation will also suffer losses."

Following the government's about-face, both *People's Daily* and *Beijing Youth News* followed suit and started to beef up their coverage of SARS. *Beijing Youth News* began to carry a "*Combating SARS*" section, which ranged from two to eight pages, on April 19, and the SARS tallies on April 21, a day earlier than *People's Daily.*

On Party and government leaders

As state-controlled media, both *People's Daily* and *Beijing Youth News* are obliged to act as mouthpieces of the Party and government. *People's Daily* kept devoting large space to the coverage of government directives and the activities of Party and state leaders. *Beijing Youth News,* on the other hand, tended to cut down the routine coverage of Party leaders and tried to find a connection between the "voice of the Party and government" and people's daily life.

When new SARS cases reached a daily record of 179 on April 26, both *People's Daily* and *Beijing Youth News* devoted much space of their front page to SARS the following day. The extensive SARS coverage on that particular day allows us to better see how the two newspapers differed in their approach to covering the Chinese leaders.

SARS was a major topic in all the eight news stories that appeared on the front page of *People's Daily*, but they all involved Party and government leaders, including the current and former Party General Secretaries, Vice-President of the state, parliament head, premier and vice premiers. It does not matter whether they were talking to foreign dignitaries or domestic audiences, they all expressed the belief that China would overcome the SARS problem through concerted efforts.

Beijing Youth News also highlighted the "voice of government," as eight out of eleven front-page stories published on that day also involved government and Party leaders. However, it chose to highlight some different stories. For example, the story on Party leader Jiang Zemin's meeting with the Indian Minister of Defense was reported in only two sentences, whereas a story about Prime Minister Wen Jiabao talking about SARS with college students over lunch was presented as the lead story of the day. Similar angles could be found in stories with headlines such as "Prime Minister Encourages Front-Line Doctors" and "Prime Minister Concerned about Teachers and Students." Unlike *People's Daily,* which featured two pictures of Chinese leaders on its first page on April 27, *Beijing Youth News* featured a couple putting up a banner to thank medical workers in a neighboring hospital.

Another example of how the two newspapers dealt with news about the leaders could be found in their coverage of a televised meeting chaired by Vice-Premier Wu Yi on April 24. In its typical fashion, *People's Daily* promptly reported the meeting the following day by giving a summary of Wu's speech and a list of VIPs attending the meeting. As an instrument to convey messages from the government, *People's Daily* performed its duty faithfully but not innovatively. *Beijing Youth News*, on the other hand, chose to report the meeting two days later. Instead of listing everything Wu said at the meeting, it chose to highlight Wu's call for the public to take precautionary measures to prevent further spread of the epidemic. In response to Wu's call, the paper also used a reader's letter, an editor's column, and pictorial caricatures to condemn certain unhealthy practices conducive to the spread of the epidemic.

In general, our reading of the news stories involving the Party and state leaders shows that both *People's Daily* and *Beijing Youth News* tended to highlight the Party and state leaders in their coverage of SARS, but *Beijing Youth News* usually cut down the coverage of routine activities and speeches of the leaders and chose to convey the "voices of government" more relevant to people's life. As a result, the leaders in *Beijing Youth News* appeared to be more humane and closer to the people. *People's Daily,* on the other hand, tended to convey the leaders' instructions regarding SARS in a timelier and more comprehensive manner without focusing on what is of relevance to the general public.

On health workers

Both newspapers covered the medical workers extensively. *People's Daily* tended to describe medical workers as role models whose heroic deeds in fighting the disease speak for the Party ideology. During the period under study, at least a dozen role models were created by *People's Daily.*

The first medical worker highlighted by *People's Daily* was Dr. Deng Lianxian, who died of SARS after being infected on duty. In addition to highlighting China's top leader Hu Jintao's mourning for the doctor, the paper carried a story entitled "Song of Life Composed by Life," in which Deng was identified as Communist Party secretary of his medical unit. In addition to what he did as a doctor for his patients, the story highlighted how he had been voted a model Communist Party member for 13 years. Yao Jilu, Deng's professor and colleague of 30 years, was quoted as saying, "He is the best one among my students. I am not a Communist Party member, but I can see the model behavior of a Party member in him." Later reports noted that Deng was named a "Revolutionary Martyr" and "Excellent Communist Party Member."

Medical workers' efforts in treating the SARS patients were often attributed by *People's Daily* to their pursuit of the communist ideology. For example, a front page story "Communist Party Members Take Lead in the Battle against SARS" on April 21 showed a picture featuring a group of doctors wearing a small but attention-catching red Party badge on their white uniform. The hospital's Party secretary was quoted as saying that most of those who volunteered to treat SARS patients face to face were Communist Party members.

On a few occasions, *People's Daily* also carried some touching stories about the medical workers. An April 25 story, for example, carried the diary of a head nurse in a Guangzhou hospital, which recorded stories of nurses who took care of the SARS patients despite family objections and who could not see their children for a long time while being quarantined in the hospital. She wrote about how she burst into tears when she heard her daughter saying on the phone, "Mummy, I miss you so much, please come back, I will not make you angry any more. You want me to sing a song for you now?" Such touching stories, however, were overshadowed by stories singing praises for medical workers inspired by the communist ideology in their fight against SARS.

Compared with *People's Daily*, *Beijing Youth News* tended to portray medical workers as ordinary people with strong commitment to their profession instead of portraying them as extraordinary people. For instance, an April 23 story focused on the daily routines of doctors in the quarantine wards, highlighting such facts as that the doctors got wet with sweat under the thick layers of protective suits and that they could not relieve themselves for hours on duty. A May 27 story, based on the letter from a SARS patient to her nurses, allowed the readers to see the medical workers through the eyes of patients.

Occasionally, *Beijing Youth News* also carried stories that related the work of health workers to political agitation. For example, a May 26 story headlined "Head Nurse Applies for Admission into Communist Party" quoted the heroine as saying that "the heroic acts of Communist Party members reinforced my wish to join the Communist Party." In an advertisement titled "Image of a Communist Party Member" on May 25, *Beijing Youth News* featured a nurse who was applying makeup to make her look better on the day she was to swear in as a Communist Party member.

Unlike *People's Daily*, which focused on singing praises for medical workers, *Beijing Youth News* tended to highlight the human interest aspect of the stories. For example, a May 14 story featured Yang Tao, a 43-year-old doctor who died after contracting SARS from his patient, with a picture showing a corner of his small home where his wife and son were sadly staring at his favorite fishing rod, with the superimposed caption "When to Go Fishing with Daddy Again." The story told how Yang's promise of buying his son a pair of new glasses had become an unfulfilled wish. The story ended with the comment, "he does not have many great achievements to speak of, but he is really a good man, a very good man."

Not all medical workers would necessarily hold their professional obligations above their personal safety, of course, but *People's Daily* chose to not report any incidence of such a nature. *Beijing Youth News*, on the other hand, carried two news stories on the dismissal of nurses who refused to join other medical workers in treating SARS patients. [See Lu, this volume, for additional examples of the role model phenomenon.]

On the public

Not much coverage was given by *People's Daily* to the general public and how their lives were affected by the epidemic. The ordinary people infrequently featured in the central Party organ were openly laden with ideological values. In fact, *People's Daily* did not carry any reports on how the epidemic was affecting people's life until May 2 when it published on the second page its first report of quarantine measures in Beijing headlined "Though under Quarantine, We Are Not Lonely," in which a SARS patient explained what the local authorities had done to make sure his daily life was in order. *Beijing Youth News,* on the other hand, devoted a large part of its coverage to the ordinary people with no political strings attached.

Beijing Youth News started to explain the quarantine measure beginning April 19, four days before its implementation. Besides introducing the quarantine experiences overseas, the paper also ran an editorial titled "Quarantine Does Not Mean Discrimination." On the first day (April 23) that Beijing put a few places under quarantine, *Beijing Youth News* rebutted the rumor that the whole city would be quarantined.

When panic buying started after the Chinese government admitted the underreporting of SARS cases on April 20, *Beijing Youth News* carried several stories on how staple food was being transported to Beijing and quoted retailers to assure readers of sufficient supply of daily necessities. *People's Daily* also reported adequate supply of goods but chose to quote Beijing government officials to assure the public instead. *Beijing Youth News* also tried to assure their readers by carrying stories about how public mailboxes, telephone booths, cash, ATMs and toilets were disinfected in the city.

According to Charity (1995), the characteristic of public journalism is to seek the community's capacity. Public listening can keep the newspaper grounded on the needs and concerns of the public. Although the concept of public journalism employed in the United States may not be applicable to China's context, the idea of public involvement is underlined by market journalism. For that purpose, *Beijing Youth News* opened a *"Hotline"* page for news items supplied by readers. On the top left corner of the page was a 24-hour hotline number. An "information fee" of 30 Chinese *yuan* was paid for each news item published. And a daily competition was organized to award best news stories with prizes ranging from 100 to 1000 *yuan*. One reader's suggestion published in the *Hotline* led to the establishment of an "Angel Fund" to reward and support medical workers and their family members. In less than a month, a total of 4,573,204 *yuan* was raised.

In addition to reporting the news, *Beijing Youth News* also attempted to get their readers directly involved in the fight against SARS. For example, it set up a 24-hour "Support Medical Workers" hotline to allow medical staff and their family members to call in for help with their family needs. Another hotline was opened to recruit volunteers who could help the medial workers and their families. When a doctor, who was quarantined in the hospital, called for tutors for her twin sons, over 50 readers volunteered their service.

People's Daily also attempted to bring the news about SARS closer to the public by running stories on ordinary people, albeit within its ideological framework. For example, a story on a taxi driver talked about how he and his wife, also a taxi driver, kept offering their service during the SARS period for public convenience. As a result, the taxi driver was allowed to join the Communist Party. By contrast, stories about the ordinary people in *Beijing Youth News* carried less political flavor.

Discussion of the findings

A country's press system invariably takes on the "the form and coloration of the social and political structures within which it operates" (Siebert, Peterson & Schramm 1963, p. 1). Therefore, it is unrealistic to expect *People's Daily* and *Beijing Youth News* to be fundamentally different in covering the SARS epidemic. Although the two newspapers may exist for different purposes, their operation is first and foremost restricted by China's overall social and political structures.

The SARS epidemic, which presented a serious threat to the life of millions of people, was by all means a news event that no media could afford to miss. Failing to report a life-and-death event would no doubt be catastrophic for an institution whose primary function is surveillance. Unfortunately, the epidemic showed the Achilles' heel of the Chinese press system. Neither *People's Daily* nor *Beijing Youth News* could break the restraints imposed by the country's political framework. Newspapers in China are, first and foremost, tools of the Communist Party and government to promote the communist ideology and state policies. When the Party and state believed that it would be best to censor the information about SARS to avoid undue panic, the press had no choice but to follow the order. Neither the efforts of individual journalists nor the power of the market could turn the tide.

In general, the coverage of SARS by both *People's Daily* and *Beijing Youth News* was consistent with the tune set by the Party and state. From the early cover-up to limited reporting later and more objective reporting in the end, both *People's Daily* and *Beijing Youth News* closely followed the Party's instructions. The dramatic changes in the two newspapers' coverage of the disease reflected the policy changes of the Party and state rather than the editorial decisions of the two newspapers. Neither the conscience of journalists nor the market demand was powerful enough to allow the newspapers to determine their own course of action.

Having said that, we must acknowledge that there were also some important differences between the two newspapers in covering the epidemic, and not all of these differences are technical in nature. First and foremost, the two newspapers seemed to differ in terms of the degree of their loyalty to their two masters – the Party and the public. Whereas *People's Daily* tried to uphold the Party line even in its coverage of the ordinary people, *Beijing Youth News* was clearly following the mass line without stepping outside the boundaries defined by the Party. For example, although *Beijing Youth News* had also failed to report the true figures of SARS cases before the government changed its cover-up strategy, it was not so difficult for its savvy readers to understand the hidden meaning of its story about the shortage of surgical masks on the market. In addition, it also highlighted the Beijing mayor's comment that the current reporting system failed to include all the SARS cases in the city in mid-April. What is more, it even quoted Dr. Jiang Yanyong to remind the Chinese society of the importance of respecting facts.

The examples above, though not directly challenging the Party's order for censorship, deviated from the official Party stand on the issue and were clearly missing in the more official *People's Daily*. Such differences could not be accounted for by differences in the training of journalists at the two newspapers because *People's Daily* tends to have better trained journalists, who are known for their challenging spirit. What made the difference must lie in the ownership and the editorial policies of the two newspapers. *People's Daily*, as an organ of the Communist Party, sees as its priority in promoting the communist ideology and state policies in its news reports. *Beijing Youth News*, on the other hand, tends to attach more importance to its readers. As long as it does not directly challenge the Party and government, it will report news in the way its readers like to see it. As a result, *Beijing Youth News* did provide, within the orbit of the Party line, some more accurate information behind the scenes even though it still fell short of being objective, especially when the truth was not what the ruling party desired.

As a central Party organ enjoying government subsidy, *People's Daily* could continue its practice of Party journalism without worrying too much about the bottom line. *Beijing Youth News*, being a financially independent but politically dependent newspaper, was facing a big dilemma in serving two masters. It could not alienate the Party, which issued its license for operation, and neither could it afford to dissatisfy its readers, who provide the financial means for its existence. For both newspapers, the Party is supreme since it could decide the fate of the newspapers as well as that of the journalists. Neither newspaper could openly defy the Party's order. For that reason, there is no significant difference between the two papers when the Party's interest is in direct conflict with the public interest. Both newspapers had to choose the Party above the public. The differences between the two newspapers would surface, however, when the Party's stance does not go directly against the public's interest. The market-oriented paper would find greater need to bring its readers more accurate and more interesting news.

It is within such a context that *Beijing Youth News* was able to find a common ground between the bottom line and the Party line by aggressively pursuing the bottom line without opposing the Party line. By blending the concept of the people who are seen as masters of the society in the theory of Party journalism with the concept of consumers who are seen as Gods in market imperatives, a commercialized press can bring some important and positive changes to the Chinese media.

Being the official newspaper of the Party, *People's Daily* obviously sees itself as a voice of the Party and state. As a result, it had to devote large space to the monotonous coverage of speeches and activities of the Party leaders and achievements of the government in the fight against SARS. When such reports dominate the coverage, it leaves little room for the creativeness of journalists, resulting in a top-down communication format.

Being a paper without such strong ties to the establishment, *Beijing Youth News* is not obligated to report everything the Party leaders said or did. While still giving prominence to the coverage of Party and government leaders, *Beijing Youth News* was given much room to convey the voices of Party and state from readers' perspective. Although its editorial staff cannot totally ignore what the Party leaders said or did, they could vary the length of stories according to their relevance to the public. Unlike *People's Daily,* which has to allocate space to the coverage of Party leaders according to their ranks, *Beijing Youth News* can more or less determine the space of coverage according to the news value of each story.

When it comes to coverage of the medical workers, the two newspapers also differed extensively. Burdened with the task of promoting the communist ideology, *People's Daily* had to provide role models to inspire other people in time of crisis. As a result, they had to present the medical workers as people imbued with the communist idea of sacrificing their own interests for the society rather than just being committed professionals and moral citizens. By contrast, *Beijing Youth News* was not obligated to portray the medical personnel as politically charged professionals. It tended to depict them as ordinary people who were performing their professional duties out of their own conscience as citizens. Not all of them were heroic fighters. Some of them could also show cowardice and decide to be derelict in their duties when their own life was threatened. More human touches were added to the portrayal of medical workers when episodes of human interest and entertainment values were included in the stories, bringing the medical workers closer to the public.

A major difference between a Party newspaper and a commercial newspaper lies in their attitude towards the public. In general, ordinary people could seldom be found in *People's Daily* stories unless they exemplify the communist ideology. Neither did *People's Daily* pay direct attention to the needs and interests of the ordinary people in its SARS coverage. In contrast, *Beijing Youth News* offered a more diversified and candid representation of the ordinary people. Noticeable efforts were made to cover the life of the public to meet their daily needs. Moreover, it also set up channels to allow its readers to have a hand in determining the news published. Its direct involvements in the fight against SARS such as its fund raising effort have brought it closer to the public, offering a sharp contrast to the stand-aloof style of Party journalism.

Conclusion

Our analysis of the SARS coverage by *People's Daily* and *Beijing Youth News* shows that the combination of Party line and bottom line determines the news today in China. The Party line, which has a long tradition in the Chinese press system, still reins supreme despite all the changes in the country's economic, political and social structures. News is still seen as a tool for the Party and state to achieve national consensus and mobilize efforts for economic development. Therefore, it can be suppressed or promoted for the interests of the Party and state as the Chinese leaders see fit.

Having said that, we must acknowledge that the bottom line does make some differences. When a newspaper like *People's Daily* receives both editorial instructions and financial support from the Party, it has little incentive to present news from a public angle. Such a newspaper is really meant for Party and government officials. A commercial newspaper, whose bottom line lies in massive circulation and high advertising rates, sees the public as its real master. The Party line, which has to be followed as a precondition for the publication of a newspaper, does not by itself provide the reason for its existence. Once the basic requirement of Party line is met, the bottom line of a commercial newspaper will drive its operation closer to the readers, whose taste and demand are more likely to be taken care of.

From a functional perspective, a commercial newspaper serves China's contemporary system better if the Chinese leaders really want the media to be "close to the fact, close to the people and close to life" as Party Secretary General Hu Jintao demanded (Zhang 2003). The bottom line of the commercial press pulls it closer to the people, who will in turn lead it closer to facts and their life. In this aspect, the structures of the press system, rather than the individual efforts of the journalists or the editorial policies of a media establishment, seem to play a more important role in determining the content of the news media in China today.

References

Charity, A. (1995). *Doing public journalism*. New York: Guilford.

Du, K. (2004). *Dancing with chains: A comparative analysis of Chinese media's coverage of the SARS crisis*. Unpublished MA thesis. Fullerton: California State University, Fullerton.

Esarey, A. W. (2006). *Caught between state and society: The commercial media in China*. Unpublished doctoral dissertation. Columbia University.

Goffman, E. (1974). *Frame analysis*. Philadelphia: University of Pennsylvania Press.

Huang, C. J. (2001). China's state-run tabloids: The rise of "city newspaper." *Gazette, 63*(5), 435–450.

Lee, C.-C. (Ed.). (1990). *Voices of China: The interplay of politics and journalism*. New York: Guilford Press

Lee, C.-C. (Ed.). (2003). *Chinese media, global contexts*. New York: Routledge.

Liu, L. (2003). *The discussion of the titles of news*. (Xinwen biaoti yantao.) Beijing: Chinese Social Science Publishing House.

Pan, Z. D. (2000). Improvising reform activities: The changing reality of journalistic practice in China. In C. C. Lee (Ed.), *Power, money, and media: Communication patterns and bureaucratic control in cultural China* (pp. 68–111). Evanston, IL: Northwestern University Press.

Pan, Z. D., & Kosicki, G. M. (1993). Framing analysis: An approach to news discourse. *Political Communication, 10*, 55–75.

Polumbaum, J. (1994). Striving for predictability: The bureaucratization of media management in China. In C. C. Lee (Ed.), *China's media, media's China* (pp. 113–128). Denver, CO: Westview.

Siebert, F. S., Peterson, T., & Schramm, W. (1963). *Four theories of the press*. Urbana: University of Illinois Press.

Tuchman, G. (1978). *Making news: A study in the construction of reality*. New York: Free Press.

World Health Organization (September 26, 2003). Summary of probable SARS cases with onset of illness from 1 November, 2002 to 31 July, 2003. Communicable Disease Surveillance & Response (CSR), World Health Organization website. Retrieved October 4, 2004 from http://www.who.int/csr/sars/country/table2003_09_23/en/.

Yu, X. (1994). Professionalization without guarantees. *Gazette, 53*, 23–41.

Zhang, W. (1997). *Politics and freedom of the press*. Sydney: Australian Centre for Independent Journalism.

Zhang, Y. (2003). Making new progress in achieving the three "closers." *News Front, 45*(5). Retrieved October 19, 2004 from http://www.people.com.cn/GB/paper79/9251/858668. html.

Zhao, Y. Z. (1998). *Media, market and democracy in China: Between the Party line and bottom line*. Urbana: University of Illinois Press.

CHAPTER 6

Construction of nationalism and political legitimacy through rhetoric of the anti-SARS campaign

A fantasy theme analysis

Xing Lu
DePaul University

Employing Ernest Bormann's (1972) fantasy theme analysis methodology, this chapter examines selected rhetorical texts and symbolic actions in the coverage of China's anti-SARS campaign. Fantasy themes of character, action, and setting are identified and analyzed. The study finds that through the positive portrayal of national leaders and the heroic acts of medical workers, a renewed sense of nationalism was constructed, characterized by patriotism and sacrifice for the Party and country. The anti-SARS rhetoric nationwide also provided moral legitimacy for the new leadership in the time of political transition. The rhetorical vision created through fantasy themes promoted a unified national spirit and reinforced the traditional Chinese cultural value of collectivism.

"萬眾一心，眾志成城，團結互助,同舟共濟，迎難而上，敢於勝利" (Unite as one; build a human wall; help each other; row in the same boat; confront the challenge; and achieve victory).

Hu Jintao's 24 words during the anti-SARS campaign.

The outbreak of SARS in spring 2003 brought China to the center of world attention. Fearing its economic and political impact, the Chinese government initially attempted to minimize the extent and danger of the SARS outbreak, thus failing to take early preventive measures to control the spread of the disease. When the cover-up fell apart,[1] the new leaders of China, President Hu Jintao and Premier

---

1. The cover-up was leaked by Dr. Jiang Yanyong of the General Hospital of the Chinese People's Liberation Army to *Time* magazine when he charged that the official statistics of SARS cases were untrue and that a large number of SARS patients were being treated in Beijing hospitals.

Wen Jiabao, exercised their authority in leading the nation against SARS.[2] They openly demanded accurate reports of SARS and ordered the removal of a number of high-ranking public officials,[3] thus, politicizing SARS at the national level. Western observers tend to consider such dramatic moves to be a victory of liberal-minded new leaders over the conservative political approach characterized by a lack of transparency in the political mindset of the old guard. However, such a move may not be simply a sign of openness or internal political struggle. The public campaign against SARS was essential for establishing the political legitimacy of the new administration and has actually generated a renewed sense of nationalism among the people.

Beginning early April 2003, the government launched a nationwide campaign against SARS. Public discourse was filled with anti-SARS slogans, patriotic sentiment, propaganda appeasing popular fears and appealing to national unity, media reports of heroic acts of medical workers, medical research achievements, visits of Hu Jintao and Wen Jiabao to various places, and images of national leaders mingling with ordinary Chinese people. Numerous newspaper articles, books, and performances were produced to promote the national spirit in overcoming the crisis.

I contend in this chapter that the Chinese discourse on SARS was consciously politicized in the government's effort to strengthen the moral authority of the new leaders. The anti-SARS rhetoric in the public domain served to promote a renewed sense of nationalism characterized by patriotism and the creation of new national heroes; it helped reinvigorate traditional Chinese cultural values of collectivism and sacrifice; and it made a case to legitimize the new leadership in the time of political transition. I will use fantasy-theme analysis to examine the rhetoric of setting, character, and action themes in the anti-SARS discourse. I will also identify the rhetorical vision created by fantasy themes that served to unite the nation, celebrate traditional Chinese culture, and exert social control.

---

2.   Hu Jintao succeeded Jiang Zemin as the Party's General Secretary in November 2002 and became the President of China in March 2003, just as the SARS crisis was beginning to catch international attention. Wen Jiabao took on the premiership at the same time.

3.   According to Chan (2003), President Hu Jintao convened a meeting of the Politburo Standing Committee of the CCP on April 7, 2003. At the meeting, Hu warned against the covering up of SARS cases and demanded a full disclosure of the epidemic. Zhang Wenkang, the Health Minister, was dismissed from office for stating at the Press conference that the disease had not reached Beijing and tourists were safe. Meng Xuenong, the Mayor of Beijing, was also removed from office for failing to take immediate measures to prevent SARS.

Chinese nationalism

While nationalism in the 19th century gave force to sovereignty and emancipation from colonial domination on a global scale, it is defined by Avraham and First (2003) as "a psychological phenomenon, involving needs and dispositions and its significance in the modern world" (p. 284). Nationalism in contemporary political context has an emotional link to national symbols, political leaders, and cultural values. The Chinese national consciousness in the early 20th century, shaped by the experience of resentment and humiliation by Western powers and the desire to modernize, led to the revolutions initially orchestrated by Dr. SunYat-sen and continued along a more radical path by Mao Zedong. According to Townsend (1996), Chinese nationalism "initially displayed a strong ethnic, even xenophobic, strain in opposing imperialism and Manchu rule" (p. 16). However, under the communist rule, nationalism is characterized by state-inculcated patriotic political appeals, Han ethnic identification, and culturalist pride (Unger 1996).

With the demise of Maoist ideology since the end of the Cultural Revolution (1966–1976), there has been an urgent need to address the "crisis of faith" and find a new base for the political legitimacy of the ruling party (Kluver 1996). McGee (1999) states, "When there is no fundamental belief, one senses a crisis which can only be met with a new rhetoric, a new mythology" (p. 347). The need for filling the ideological vacuum requests new types of discourse to strengthen the political legitimacy (Simons 1970).

The regimes of the post-Mao period have embraced nationalism as the new base of legitimacy to sustain the party rule. Leaders of the new regimes have presented themselves as the guardians of national pride in national and international contexts. Nationalism has become a new mythology replacing Marxist-Maoist revolutionary ideology and to serve as a rhetorical strategy to unite the nation. Zheng (1999) has observed that "The [current] official discourse of nationalism has focused on patriotism" (p. 88). Chang (2001) concurred with this observation by giving the example of the Patriotic Education Campaign in 1995. They both agree that Chinese nationalism is facilitated by the discourse of loyalty and sacrifice to the state. Through examining public discourse on patriotism, Chang (2001) identified aspects of "Chinese spirit" that includes "patriotism, industriousness, perseverance, achievement, collectivism, and revolutionary enthusiasm" (p. 183). This list, although claimed as "communist sentiments and principles" indicated an appropriation of traditional Chinese cultural values as promoted and taught by Confucian doctrines. The public discourse in the anti-SARS campaign exhibited the types of patriotic discourse, featuring collectivism, perseverance, sacrifice, national pride in the forms of narrative, media images, letters, diaries, and speeches.

Methodology: The fantasy-theme analysis

Fantasy theme analysis is a method of rhetorical criticism aimed at discovering recurring communication patterns in the interpretation and evaluation of rhetorical texts and symbolic actions. Fantasy is defined as "the creative and imaginative shared interpretation of events that fulfils a group psychological or rhetorical need" (Bormann 1985, p. 130). The method was derived from Robert Bales' (1970) observation on small group communication in which group members grow excited and emotional, laughing, cajoling, and dramatizing a situation, a character, or an action through the process of their verbal and nonverbal interactions. According to Ernest Bormann (1983), a fantasy-theme analysis identifies patterns of human interaction and analyzes how these patterns serve to construct and reconstruct realities for individuals and groups in their participation in a rhetorical experience.

The method was developed by Bormann based on his symbolic convergence theory. In Bormann's words (1985), "The theory explains the appearance of a group consciousness, with its implied shared emotions, motives, and meanings, not in terms of individual day dreams and scripts but rather in terms of socially shared narrations or fantasies" (p. 128). Basically, the theory claims that in the process of communication, participants jointly create a drama or an emotionally charged experience resulting in a convergence of meanings. The outcome of this convergence is a new sense of reality guiding participants' perceptions and behaviours in social contexts. The method has been applied to the study of small group communication as well to the study of media, advertising, political debates, social movements, as well as ritualistic practices (e.g. Foss 1979; Foss & Littlejohn 1986; Garner, Sterk, & Adams 1998; Putman, Van Hoeven, & Bullis 1991).

In his own application of the method, Bormann discovered that group members often create narratives that contain dramatic descriptions of heroes, heroines, and villains. Hence, fantasy is created in a way similar to how a drama is played out, involving elements of scene, character, and action. Bormann classified fantasy themes, then, as character themes, action themes, and setting themes. *Character themes* describe the actors who are portrayed as heroes or villains in the drama, including their qualities and motives. *Action themes* refer to the actions performed by the characters in the drama. *Setting themes* depict the places or scenes where actions take place. Bormann and his colleagues (2003) contend that these elements of rhetorical fantasies are discoverable through fantasy-theme analysis. Further, "They can be translated because meaning, emotion, value, and motive for action are present in the communication" (p. 368).

When fantasy themes are shared by group members or mass media audiences, a common ground for communication is created. Group members or mass media audiences would consider certain characters as heroes or villains and regard certain actions as laudable or undesirable. This shared consciousness will lead to the construction of a rhetorical vision for a rhetorical community. A *rhetorical vision* is "a unified putting together of the various scripts that give the participants a broader view of things" (Bormann 1983, p. 133). In other words, it is "a swirling together of fantasy themes to provide a particular interpretation of reality" (Foss 2004, p. 112). A rhetorical vision is usually indexed by a set of key words or slogans. For example, current slogans for the rhetorical vision in the United States are "anti-terrorism," "homeland security." When a rhetorical vision is shared by a rhetorical community through fantasies or "dramatizing messages," people will begin to think and act based on a mutual understanding of the reality in which they participate. The convergence of symbolic meanings takes place, calling for a common sense of purpose, motivation, and action.

In this chapter, I will use fantasy-theme analysis to uncover how a patriotic reality is constructed through character, action, and setting themes, and describe how a rhetorical vision is created in promoting nationalism and legitimizing the political rule in contemporary China. The rhetorical data analyzed include books documenting the nationwide fight against SARS as well as reports from the *People's Liberation Army (PLA) Daily* covering the topic. All the books were published in 2003 during and after the SARS campaign and written by Chinese authors who are professional reporters, editors, or writers.[4] The process of the analysis involves two steps: (1) coding the rhetorical texts for setting, character, and action themes; (2) constructing the rhetorical vision from the fantasy themes (Foss 2004).

Identification of fantasy themes

This section will analyze the character, action, and setting themes located in the data.

---

4. There are no exact figures on how many books were published during the anti-SARS campaign in China. I, however, purchased the six books I could find in bookstores of Beijing on the topic of SARS in the summer of 2003 and most of them are referenced in this chapter. The publishers are all from Mainland China. There are many similar newspaper reports on the anti-SARS campaign in China. The books I referenced contained widely published reports and events taking place during this time period from in China's media.

Character themes

Two character themes are identified from the rhetorical texts being examined. The first focuses largely on political leaders, mainly Hu Jintao and Wen Jiabao, who were portrayed in the media as being in the forefront of the campaign and having exhibited the qualities of care and compassion for the Chinese people. The second character theme is centered around medical workers, largely doctors and nurses who played indispensable roles in the control and treatment of SARS. They were portrayed as loyal, unselfish, courageous, and heroic.

New political leaders as confident, compassionate, and competent

Hu Jintao, the President of China, and Wen Jiabao, China's Premier, are the new generation of leaders, succeeding Jiang Zemin and Zhu Rongji in the spring of 2003. Although Jiang resigned from the positions of China's President and the CCP's (Chinese Communist Party) General Secretary, he was still the commander in chief in the military, the real power behind the scene at the time of the SARS epidemic. Hu and Wen were not considered Jiang's loyalists and it was suspected that the initial cover-up of SARS was instructed by Jiang. Hu and Wen would have risked their political career if they had openly declared defiance against Jiang before their election by allowing accurate reports of the spread of SARS to appear. Further, as they were still new leaders, they faced the challenge of establishing their leadership credibility among the Chinese people.

Despite the political pressure, Hu and Wen emerged in public with assertiveness and became the most frequently portrayed characters in the media and public discourse after the SARS cover-up was exposed. In *Reports of SARS* (Yu 2003), Hu was described as coming to Guangzhou (the city where the first case of SARS was found) on April 14th, 2003, and visiting the Provincial Disease Control Center. He talked with doctors and nurses from twenty-three branches of the medical center and solicited information about the SARS prevention campaign. The book reports that Hu did not wear a face mask while talking with doctors and nurses, suggesting that he was not afraid of contracting SARS and sending a message to the Chinese people that there was nothing to fear. Later in the evening, Hu came to the busiest street in Guangzhou, stepping out of his car and shaking hands with ordinary people (pp. 191–192).

In the same source, Premier Wen was reported to have come to Guangzhou on April 30th. He first visited a middle school, then walked around a few stores. Like Hu, Wen shook hands with people on the street and chatted with them freely, which was not scheduled as part of the agenda. Nantie Xu (2003), author of the book, commented, "Facing the crisis of SARS, China's new leaders demonstrated their style and confidence" (p. 192). Similar praise can be found in Lin's (2003) *Wall of People: Chinese People's Fight Against SARS*.

> The new leaders always keep cool headed and have a strong sense of concern for China. Because of these qualities, they are aware of the seriousness of the SARS epidemic. They are calm and well organized. They quickly mobilized all resources and led Chinese people in fighting against SARS.   (p. 25)

Such a portrayal of Chinese leaders (character theme) greatly enhanced the perceived competence of the new leaders and altered the negative image of China from the initial cover-up on SARS.

The book by Lin also reported the symbolic actions of people-orientation demonstrated by Hu and Wen. It describes Hu's visits to medical research centers and hospitals in Beijing, thanking scientists and medical personnel for their research contribution and encouraging them to face the crisis with confidence and determination. Lin (2003) also reports that Hu signed many executive orders endorsing specific actions to prevent SARS from spreading. The book includes a picture of Hu greeting scientists and medical personnel with a genuine smile and a gesture of hands folding together (a traditional Chinese greeting) in thanking the medical personnel. Such an act by a Chinese leader has rarely been seen in the public. Moreover, the book shows how passionate the Chinese leaders are toward their people. For example, it reports that Wen Jiabao had tears in his eyes while visiting daycare centers in Beijing. Premier Wen is reported to have been so concerned with the SARS epidemic that he could not sleep at night. Wen was quoted as saying that "A responsible government must put the interest of people first" (p. 32). The book specifically describes Premier Wen's visit to Beijing University on April 26: his having meals with students, learning about the prevention of SARS, and telling students to take care of their health. The book cited one anecdote of Premier Wen's visit to Tsinghua University on May 4th.

> While he was giving a speech on prevention of SARS, Premier Wen felt thirsty. He asked 'Who can offer me some water?' A student gave him his own mug and the Premier drank the water from it without hesitation [indicating Wen was not afraid of contracting SARS]. Students were very touched by this act. They saw a people's premier who loves his people. This gives them confidence and trust in the government.   (p. 34)

Such stories about national leaders are a powerful means of enticing the Chinese people's imagination to accept their leaders as benevolent, the type of leaders that are rhetorically constructed in Confucian works, and also portrayed during Mao Zedong's era prior to the economic reform (1949–1976).

New Chinese leaders are not only shown as caring and compassionate, but also as competent and decisive in combating SARS. The *PLA Daily* reported, "Chinese Premier Wen Jiabao set out ten tasks in the battle against severe acute respiratory syndrome (SARS), calling for improved control and prevention efforts and closer cooperation with overseas health organizations" (April 28, 2003). Some aspects of these tasks include quarantine efforts in public transportation, utilizing scientific resources at home and abroad, offering free medical service to poor patients in rural areas, and close cooperation with world health organizations. The *PLA Daily* cited the Premier as saying, "China is confident in winning over the disease and putting SARS under control, for China had the strong leadership of the Central Committee of the Communist Party and the support of the general public" (*The PLA Daily*, April 28th, 2003). The new leaders not only set out tasks, but also made sure the tasks were executed and promises were delivered. They appointed Wu Yi, the Vice Premier, to head the National SARS Control and Prevention Headquarters so that the number of SARS cases were reported every day in newspapers throughout China.

In sum, the character theme of political leaders is lofty and laudable. These reports portrayed the new Chinese leaders as humble, respectful, compassionate, caring for the people, having the competency in handling the crisis, and being capable of leading the nation. Further, they were portrayed as open, decisive and courageous as they publicly demanded a full disclosure and a stront commitment to telling the truth in dealing with SARS to the Chinese people and the world. Wen Jiabao was portrayed as having a soft heart and a good understanding of what the people and country need. "Putting People First" has been the slogan used in many of Hu and Wen's speeches. Hu and Wen's handling of SARS crisis portrayed them as applying this slogan into practice.

Medical workers as courageous, sacrificing, and patriotic

Another group of characters who took the headlines of the media are doctors and nurses who worked in hospitals saving lives of SARS patients. Many doctors and nurses were reported as heroes or heroines. Two of them stand out. One is a doctor named Zhong Nanshan, who had not only saved many lives and finally contracted SARS himself, but who also publicly cautioned the government that SARS had not been brought totally under the control and proclaimed that the truth must be told to the Chinese people and the world. He was the first person who requested international assistance for China's situation when such a move might have been perceived as denigrating the nation's pride. He was also the first person seeking collaboration with Hong Kong University in the prevention of SARS. When he was interviewed by the *Face to Face* program on TV and asked, "Do you care about politics?" his answer was "Doing my job and doing it well is politics" (Xu 2003, p. 130). Xu (2003) wrote, "During the days of fighting against SARS, Zhong Nanshan represented science and righteousness. He represented the conscience of Chinese intellectuals. When he came out in the public, he could calm down the audience, win the trust of the international community, and give the nation confidence" (p. 126). The stories of Zhong Nanshan have been published all over China and he ultimately became a national hero.

Ye Xin, the head nurse of Chinese Medical Hospital in Guangdong Province, is another hero reported widely in the media. While Ye Xin was taking care of a SARS patient, she would not let other nurses come into the ward so that the chance of contracting SARS could be reduced for others. One report says about her deeds:

> Every night after she got home, she would boil a big pot of Chinese medicine for her co-nurses for SARS prevention. During her twenty-two years of marriage, she spent every Chinese New Year in the hospital except one time. After taking care of so many SARS patients, Ye Xin contracted the deadly disease. While she was being treated, she wrote on a piece of paper "Do not come close to me. You may also get infected." Ye Xin passed away on March 24th. She was honored as a national martyr.   (Xu 2003, pp. 141–143)

Many stories were told about doctors and nurses who sacrificed their lives to save the lives of others. A collection of fifty-six letters by doctors and nurses to their families was published. All these letters expressed one common message: It is our duty as doctors and nurses to work in the front of fighting against SARS and curing SARS patients. Fighting against SARS is a life-death battle. Patients need us and we must fight till we win the battle. It is glorious to sacrifice for the country (Yu 2003).

During the anti-SARS campaign, doctors and nurses are portrayed as new heroes and heroines in China. They possess the qualities of honesty, sacrifice, perseverance, collectivism, and enthusiasm in helping others and the nation in the time of crisis. They are considered as having exemplified the "Chinese spirit" and "national character." From Confucian teachings to Maoist doctrines, role-modeling has been encouraged to promote moral ideals and character building (Munro 1977; Zhang 1999, 2000). The character theme of doctors and nurses portrayed in these books helped promote the national sentiment and cultural pride.

Action themes

Two action themes are identified in the texts being examined: the theme of *heroic and patriotic acts*, and the theme of *political and communist acts*. These action themes not only celebrated the cultural values of sacrifice, collectivism, loyalty, but they also politicized the anti-SARS campaign to legitimize the communist rule and its moral authority.

Anti-SARS activities as heroic and patriotic acts

Treating hospitals as battlefields, many doctors and nurses are portrayed as performing patriotic acts to save the nation. They petitioned for going to the "battlefield" and said tearful goodbyes to their families. An account from *Eyewitness of Xiao Tang Shan* described the scene: "Groups of marching troops were carried to the front [of the battlefield] by buses, trains, and airplanes; many unselfish emotions were expressed through petitions and letters and determination" (Jiang et al. 2003, p. 5). One story tells of a nurse who was worried about her mother while she was on her way to the battlefield. But when she called home, her mother said to her calmly, "do not worry. You have my blessings from the rear base [of the battlefield]" (p. 5). The book shows pictures of nurses and doctors in army uniforms standing in front of the hospital, an action theme that conveys a total devotion to the nation at the sacrifice of family and self.

Medical workers, especially party members, were described as the most unselfish and courageous fighters in this battle. Doctors and nurses who contracted the disease and died were described as "falling down in the battlefield." When some medical workers were asked to take a break or go home for a rest after working for long hours, the reply was, "I am a soldier in a battle; I would be a deserter from war if I leave" (Lin 2003, p. 118). In *Wall of People*, a picture shows a group of doctors taking an oath with a banner at their backs saying "Declare a war on SARS; party members are in the front" (p. 128).

Lin (2003) reported that in the most difficult and most dangerous times of the SARS battle, party members always volunteered first to go to "the front." Those who contracted the disease or died because of it were all party members. A doctor was quoted saying, "I am a party member. I must go first. This is the critical moment of combating SARS. As a party member and doctor, I absolutely cannot leave the SARS battlefield. Otherwise, I am not a party member, nor qualified as a doctor" (p. 128). As recorded in all these books, many doctors and nurses asked for "battle" assignments. Like in a regular war, brave soldiers were rewarded. Xinhua, China's official News Agency (July 18, 2003), reported that a host of people and organizations in the sciences and technology were given awards for their outstanding performance in fighting SARS. Thus, the fight against SARS was linked to the mission of the CCP and the pride of the nation. Using patriotic and nationalist appeals by top leaders has served as an organizing and mobilizing force in the battle against SARS.

Anti-SARS activities as political and communist acts
Another action theme is illustrated by showing loyalty to the CCP. The action of joining the party in "the battlefield" is reported frequently in the texts. Joining the party is a political act of showing allegiance to the party and loyalty to the country. A nationalistic spirit was greatly boosted through such an action theme. In *Eyewitness of Xiao Tang Shan*, a diary entry is included:

> Today is the most unforgettable day in my life. I proudly joined the Chinese Communist Party. . . . In the battle against SARS, I will use the criteria of party members to guide my thought and action, willing to give and sacrifice. . . . As long as we can win this battle, I voluntarily sacrifice my youth and energy. I raised my right hand and took an oath: "Strive for communism for the rest of my life."
> (Jiang et al. 2003, p. 65)

Similar scenes of taking an oath to join the Communist Party are reported in many other publications on SARS as well. One picture in *Wall of People: Chinese People's Fight Against SARS* shows that three medical personnel joined the party in their medical uniform. "Join the party in the anti-SARS front and experience the test of life and death" was a slogan during the SARS prevention period. It is reported in the book that in Beijing alone, 1,800 people joined the party within a month; many were doctors and nurses. This number is significant because the CCP has been losing its credibility among Chinese people because of the rampant corruption cases since the economic reform. Such action of massive increase in party membership indicates continued faith in the party leadership among the new heroes and helps boost the party's legitimacy. As attested by an applicant to the party:

> Within a week since I came to the SARS battlefield, I truly feel the vulnerability of life and health. I feel even more strongly about the responsibilities of doctors. . . . As a doctor, I feel proud to serve the country and people when I am most needed. This unforgettable experience also strengthened my belief in the Chinese Communist Party.
> (Lin 2003, p. 137)

The above action themes exemplified patriotic and political nature of the anti-SARS campaign. They portray the Communist Party as the unifying force for the national image and becoming a member as a personal satisfaction, reinforcing the legitimacy of party leadership and nationalist sentiments.

Setting themes

Two setting themes emerged in the texts: the physical setting of hospitals and the symbolic setting of the national "war" against SARS. The setting themes illustrated

China's technological ability to handle the crisis and the leaders' determination to win the war at the social and psychological levels.

Hospitals as the heroic setting

Several settings were portrayed in the texts such as hospitals, quarantine centers, research institutes, and press conferences or TV interviews during the anti-SARS campaign.[5] This analysis will focus on only the most frequent setting of the anti-SARS campaign: hospitals or medical centers where doctors and nurses work to save the lives of SARS patients. These hospitals were equipped with modern technology and abundant medical resources. Quarantine centers were set up all over China, the biggest one being located in Xiao Tang Shan, an outskirt of Beijing. Providing some pictures of hospital beds and medical equipment, the book *Eyewitness of Xiao Tang Shan* reported the glorious deeds in building the hospital and recorded the heroic deeds of combating SARS on the site (Jiang et al. 2003).

The order to build a special hospital for SARS patients came directly from the Military Commission of the Central Committee of the Communist Party, and a special team was formed to take charge of this task. "This is a battle of storm fortifications." Jiang and his colleagues (2003) report, "They [workers] were given five days to build 1,000 hospital beds and office space for 1,200 medical workers dispatched from hospitals in Beijing and nearby areas. . . However, in the spirit of uniting as one and forging a human wall, what seemed impossible became reality" (Jiang et al. 2003, pp. 1–2). Such descriptions of this physically setting sends the message of how unified and determined Chinese people are in fighting against SARS.

Symbolic setting: China at "war" against SARS

Apart from the creation of a physical setting theme, the symbolic setting theme was also significant in the portrayal of the anti-SARS campaign. The symbolic setting theme mentioned most frequently and with greatest intensity is the "battlefield of SARS" metaphor. A war metaphor was also used pervasively in the propaganda against SARS. From the beginning of the campaign, President Hu called for a "People's War" against SARS, with SARS being the enemy and doctors and nurses being the fighters. Hospitals and quarantine centers were referred as "battlefields without smoke." Any new cases of SARS were referred to as an "enemy situation." At a press conference, the acting mayor of Beijing used a traditional Chinese saying, "No joking matter in war" and acted as the commander in chief in the combat

---

5.   The press conferences are usually conducted in Beijing with local officials answering questions from national and international media. The interviews include officials of the World Health Organization and high profile figures of Chinese nationals during the anti-SARS battle.

battle against SARS in Beijing. The weapon to win the war is science and technology. As Hu was quoted saying, "The key to defeating the epidemic lies in bringing into play the important role of science and technology" (The *PLA Daily*, May 2, 2003). All these symbolic setting themes created during the anti-SARS campaign point to a renewed sense of national spirit and regained confidence of the CCP in leading the nation in the time of crisis.

The scientific capability to combat SARS was linked to the ability of the nation and national leaders. As Wen Jiabao reiterated, "Under the strong leadership of the Communist Party of China and the government, with abundant material and technological support, the nation is sure to achieve complete success in the battle" (*The People's Liberation Army Daily*, May 6, 2003). To win this nation-wide battle, doctors and nurses were encouraged to show "patriotic spirit" in the "battlefield." In fact, the whole campaign against SARS is referred to as a nationwide patriotic public health campaign. Wu Yi, director of the National Committee for the Patriotic Public Health Campaign, has said in many public settings that "The Chinese government is confident and capable of controlling and eradicating SARS" (*The People's Liberation Army Daily*, April 10, 2003).

Construction of rhetorical vision

Using the fantasy theme analysis, this study has examined the character, action, and setting themes in selected texts reporting SARS prevention and treatment on a nation-wide scale in China. The character and action themes appear to be the major themes of this analysis. The portrayal of the compassionate and competent images of national leaders and the patriotic/heroic acts of the medical workers engendered a revival of nationalism characterized by patriotism, sacrifice, and collectivism in the time of moral decline as the result of the economic reform since late 1970s. Seemingly, hospitals or "battlefields" provided settings for these heroic acts to take place and national leaders to perform their leadership roles. At the political level, such settings also have the symbolic meaning of engaging a national war led by new leaders and the Communist Party against both the SARS disease and the institutional disease (concealing the truth from the public). The analyses of the fantasy themes demonstrated a process of symbolic convergence that resulted in a unified rhetorical vision: **a renewed sense of nationalism and political legitimacy of the national leaders.**

This rhetorical vision has the following implications: First, the renewed nationalism is a rhetorical construction. The action themes portrayed the spirit of courage, sacrifice, and patriotism exhibited by doctors and nurses. To win or lose the war against SARS does not simply mean how many SARS patients will be cured, but how China would be perceived in the world through the exposure of these images. The frequent appearance of national leaders in various contexts in close contacts with Chinese people, along with the remarks they made showing concern for the people and expressing confidence in winning the "war" all served to strengthen the image of China as a unified and unbeatable nation. Moreover, the renewed nationalism is tied closely with renewed loyalty to the Communist Party, giving the party not only the legitimacy to rule, but also the moral authority of the nation.

Second, the renewed nationalism is promoted through the frequent appearance of national leaders among ordinary citizens, showing their concern for people, their decisive leadership, and their commitment to bring SARS under control. The new leaders put their political careers on the line both by allowing open publicity of SARS developments and also by removal of Jiang's trusted officials. Their success in leading the nation to combat SARS, and their symbolic actions of "putting people first," have given them moral legitimacy as the new generation of Chinese leaders; and they have built confidence among Chinese people. The portrayal of the political leaders characterized them as exhibiting traditional Chinese values and meeting the expectations for cultural heroes and national leaders, an image in stark contrast with those corrupt officials and new bureaucrats growing in large numbers since the economic reform.

According to Mencius (390–305 B.C.), the legitimacy of a government rests on being benevolent to and caring for its people (Menzi, Book 1, chapter 7). Benevolent rulers must have virtues and a heart of compassion, unable to bear seeing human suffering. The character portrayal of Hu and Wen presented them as such virtuous leaders, placing people's interest above everything else. According to Burke (1969), rhetoric can induce agreement and cooperation through identification, or sharing the same substance. By appealing to traditional Chinese ideals on the relationship between the people and the ruler, Hu and Wen appeared to have gained their political legitimacy and consolidated their new regime. This is expressed through the praise and expression of faith in the new leaders in the construction of the character theme in the books I examined. Through endorsement of national leaders, a national pride was boosted.

Third, the character themes portrayed in the medical workers created new heroes and heroines in Chinese culture. Model exemplars have been used from ancient to present times as a means of moral persuasion to reinforce cultural values of sacrifice and loyalty to the Chinese state, as well as to values of perseverance and collective orientation (Zhang 1999). New heroes and their spirit of sacrifice were also in direct response to the moral decline and tendency toward self-interest and a materialistic orientation among the Chinese since the economic reform (Zhang 2000). The heroes were portrayed as representing the national spirit and being patriotic to the nation. This national spirit was well expressed by doctors and nurses taking their oath to join the party and their unselfish acts in the battle against SARS.

Fourth, the rhetorical vision of renewed nationalism created through the fantasy themes exemplified the emotional characteristics of the use of symbols in the global context. In the case of China, such an emotional characteristic is patriotic in nature, with appeals to moral authority and cultural pride. This type of nationalism is needed for nations like China that have lost the ideological appeals of Mao's regime and moved to a more pragmatic orientation and individualistic culture (Lu 1998). It is also needed for the new leaders to secure their power and exercise their control. The propagation of anti-SARS rhetoric may induce the Chinese people to a collective fantasy or political myths of the new government in the fashion of an ideological commitment to nationalism. Even though McGee (1999) cautions that political myths "represent nothing but a false consciousness," he admits that these myths "nonetheless function as a means of providing social unity and collective identity" (p. 348). Anti-SARS rhetoric in the Chinese context has served such a purpose under the new generation of leaders.

References

Avraham, E., & First, A. (2003). "I buy American": The American image as reflected in Israeli advertising. *Journal of Communication, 53*, 115–132.

Bales, R. F. (1970). *Personality and interpersonal behavior.* New York: Holt, Rinehart, and Winston.

Bormann, E. G. (1972). Fantasy and rhetorical vision: The rhetorical criticism of social reality. *Quarterly Journal of Speech, 68*, 288–303.

Bormann, E. G. (1985). Symbolic convergence theory: A communication formulation. *Journal of Communication, 35*, 128–138.

Bormann, E. G., Cragan, J. F., & Shields, D. G. (2003). Defending symbolic convergence theory from an imaginary Gunn. *Quarterly Journal of Speech, 89*, 366–372.

Burke, K. (1969). *A rhetoric of motives.* Berkeley: University of California Press.

Chan, J. (2003). SARS epidemic triggers political crisis in China. WSWS: News & Analysis: China. www.wsws.org/articles/2003/may2003/sars-m03.shtml.

Chang, M. H. (2001). *Return of the dragon: China's wounded nationalism.* Boulder, CO: Westview Press.

Foss, S. (2004). *Rhetorical criticism: Exploration & practice* (3rd ed.). Long Grove, IL: Waveland Press.

Garner, A., Sterk, H. M., & Adams, S. (1998). Narrative analysis of sexual etiquette in teenage magazines. *Journal of Communication, 48*, 59–78.

Jiang, W. et al. 江宛柳 (2003). 目擊小湯山 [*Eyewitness of Xiao Tang Shan*]. Beijing: Long March Press.

Kluver, A. R. (1996). *Legitimating the Chinese economic reforms: A rhetoric of myth and orthodoxy.* Albany: State University of New York Press.

Lin, L. et al. 林路明 (2003). 眾志成城頌: 中國人民抗擊非典紀實 [*Wall of People: Chinese People's Fight Against SARS*]. Beijing: Xuexi Publication.

Lu, X. (1998). An interface between individualistic and collectivistic orientations in Chinese cultural values and social relations. *The Howard Journal of Communication, 9*, 91–107.

McGee, M. C. (1999). In search of 'the people': A rhetorical alternative. In J. L. Lucaites, C. M. Condit, & S. Caudill (Eds.), *Contemporary rhetorical theory: A reader* (pp. 341–356). New York: Guilford.

Menzi. (1992). 孟子白話今譯 [The Translation of Mencius. Li Shuang (Ed.). Beijing: China Books.

Munro, D. J. (1977). *The concept of man in contemporary China.* Ann Arbor: University of Michigan Press.

Simons, H. W. (1970). Requirements, problems, and strategies: A theory of persuasion for social movements. *Quarterly Journal of Speech, 56*, 1–11.

Townsend, J. (1996). Chinese nationalism. In J. Unger (Ed.), *Chinese nationalism* (pp. 1–30). Armonk, NY: M. E. Sharpe.

Unger, J. (1996). Introduction. In J. Unger, *Chinese nationalism* (pp. xi–xviii). Armonk, NY: M. E. Sharpe.

Xu, N. 徐南鐵 (2003). 非典的典型報告 [*Reports of SARS*]. Guangdong: Guangdong People's Press.

Yu, W., et al. 餘煒 (2003). 來自抗擊非典一線的 56 封家書 [*56 family letters from the front of SARS battlefield*]. Beijing: Life, Reading, and New Knowledge Books.

Zhang, M. (1999). From Lei Feng to Zhang Haidi: Changing media images of model youth in the post-Mao reform era. In R. Kluver & J. H. Powers (Eds.), *Civic discourse, civil society, and Chinese communities* (pp. 111–123). Stamford, CT: Ablex.

Zhang, M. (2000). Official role models and unofficial responses: Problems of model emulation in post-Mao China. In D. R. Heisey (Ed.), *Chinese perspectives in rhetoric and communication* (pp. 67–85). Stamford, CT: Ablex.

Zheng, Y. (1999). *Discovering Chinese nationalism in China: Modernization, identity, and international relations.* Cambridge: Cambridge University Press.

CHAPTER 7

SARS discourse as an anti-SARS ideology

The case of Beijing

Hailong Tian
Tianjin University of Commerce

This study examines a series of SARS case reports produced by the News Office of China's Health Ministry between 21 April and 20 May 2003. The study first examines the change of "stages" in the generic structure of the 30 case reports, and then relates these changes to the way in which the News Office selectively included and excluded SARS case information. It is observed that, by adding and deleting stages in the case reports, the News Office attached more prominence to information that went with the interests and beliefs of its own group and downgraded information that was inconsistent with their interests and desires. Preference for some information and ignoring of other information are seen as a way of representing the anti-SARS social practice and constituting the group's particular anti-SARS ideology.

Introduction

The first half of 2003 witnessed a widespread outbreak of SARS in most parts of China. The situation reached its most serious point in the second half of April, when the number of patients in Beijing became so great that hospitals seemed unable to provide them with effective treatment. What was worse, increasing numbers of doctors and nurses were infected and became patients themselves.

This situation attracted the attention of the country's senior leaders, who took several measures to curb the epidemic. For example, the government developed regulations to direct the fight against SARS in accordance with the law. It also organized a committee, with Vice Premier Wu Yi as the head, to streamline the use of available resources. With SARS being added to the list of epidemic diseases, all travelers, whether on planes, trains or coaches, were monitored to prevent SARS from spreading further. Both the central and local governments spent billions of Chinese *yuan* treating patients with both traditional Chinese medicine and modern scientific research. Due to these measures, the spread of SARS slowed within a month. On 20 May the number of newly-reported patients in Beijing decreased to 12, compared with the 145 newly-reported cases on 21 April. On 24 June, the World Health Organization (WHO) announced the removal of Beijing from its list of SARS-infected areas and lifted its travel advisory on the city.

Many actions initiated by the government contributed to the effective control of the SARS epidemic. One such measure was that SARS cases from all areas of the country were reported to the public daily by the News Office of the Ministry of Health. The reporting began on 21 April and continued in the following months. On the first few days, the case briefings occurred at different times of the day, but they were soon regularly held at 4 pm and made public by various news media. The SARS cases were originally presented in the form of a statistical diagram, which simply contained objective case numbers. The News Office then turned the objective numbers into a daily case report in the form of text, which evolved over time to produce a series of case reports.

Thirty of these SARS case reports, produced between 21 April and 20 May 2003, were chosen as data for this study. They will be examined in terms of changes in their generic structure, a type of textual structure that resembles a sequence of speech acts in achieving the communicator's discursive purposes. Based on a theoretical premise drawn from critical discourse analysis (CDA) that discourse may function as an expression of social practice, changes in the generic structure of these case reports over time will be analyzed to discover how the News Office represented the fight against SARS, by either including or excluding certain SARS case information at various times. The study indicates that the News Office attached more prominence to information that went with the interests and beliefs of its sponsoring group (i.e., officials of the Ministry of Health) and downgraded information that was inconsistent with their interests and desires. The shifting preference for including some information while ignoring other information in the SARS case reports is identififed as the group's *anti-SARS ideology*. The following two sections first spell out the theoretical premise upon which this study is based and then explain the tool it adopts to analyze changes in the generic structure of the case reports.

Theoretical premise: Discourse and the anti-SARS ideology

A group's ideology is expressed in the discourse it produces – that is, the choice of topics it discusses and how its encodes in language the ways it talks about them. Moreover, the concept of an ideology is frequently treated in terms of the power relations that exist in society and the language used to promote or resist them. Especially prominent is concern with questions related to whose discourse and interests are influential in guiding a society's actions and whose are effectively marginalized. In the society of late modernity, where a powerful group is more likely to influence people's minds than to restrain their actual freedom of action, power is often exercised through the control of the discursive practices that are encouraged or discouraged.

Because ideologies are embedded in routine text and talk, they are often implicit, misperceived as being natural rather than arbitrary, and accepted as legitimate without inquiring into the alternatives. It is here that CDA becomes particularly relevant because CDA may be used to denaturalize the ideologies upon which the orderliness of interaction depends (Fairclough 1985) and demystify the discourse by deciphering the underlying ideologies (Wodak 2001). According to van Dijk (1993, 1995, 1998, 1999), the power and ideology that represent social structure are expressed in discourse structure through the dominant producer's control of access to both the context in which discourse is produced and the discourse itself.

Accordingly, the SARS case reports in this study are taken as ideologically significant discourse because they reveal the Ministry of Health's SARS social practice (Fairclough 2003; van Leeuwen 1993). This is important because there are competing ways in which SARS social practice might be represented. For example, SARS could have been represented as a formidable disaster for human beings, thereby fostering an overwhelming pessimistic atmosphere; or it could have been seen as an inspiring impetus, thereby encouraging people to fight against the epidemic with a positive spirit. In the current context, the SARS case reports represent the social practice in a way that helps fight against the SARS epidemic. In this sense, these SARS case reports constitute a particular type of "anti-SARS ideology" that favors the government's approach to fighting against the SARS epidemic. Just as ideologies "are the fundamental social cognitions that reflect the basic aims, interests and values of groups" (van Dijk 1993, p. 113), the Ministry of Health's anti-SARS ideology is a particular way of representing the SARS cases in language that helped the government fight against the SARS epidemic in the particular way it chose.

To elaborate the point concerning ideology and power, we can turn to van Dijk (1993), who identifies several strategies that producers can apply to control access to communication context and the discourse produced within it. In terms of the context of communication, for example, the dominant producer may control access to the occasion, time, place, and setting; the presence or absence of certain participants in the events; the modes of participation; the overall organization of the event, and the news media who report the event. Each contextual factor contributes to how recipients of the discourse are likely to understand what is normal social practice.

In terms of the actual discourse produced in the contexts provided, the dominant producer may control access to such things as the topics, style, genre, agenda, turn taking, marginalization or exclusion of some "voices," and the withholding of certain information. Thus, in van Dijk's (1993) terms, the core of critical discourse analysis involves "a detailed description, explanation and critique of the ways dominant discourses (indirectly) influence such socially shared knowledge, attitudes and ideologies, namely through their role in the manufacture of concrete models" (p. 114) that people use to interpret their personal and social experience. Starting from this point, the present study examines how the News Office exercised its control over the actual discourse of SARS, as presented in the textual structure of its case reports. Issues related to their control of the contextual issues are only implicitly mentioned where they are relevant, but they are not given explicit analysis in this chapter.

Analytical tool: Generic structure analysis

At the micro level where the actual discourse of SARS was produced by the Ministry of Health's News Office, we shall concentrate our analysis on the textual structure of the case reports presented. At this level, the analytical tool adopted is *generic structure analysis*, which is based on systemic functional linguistics (SFL). In generic structure analysis, a discourse genre consists of "diverse ways of acting, of producing social life, in the semiotic mode" (Fairclough 2001, p. 235). Eggins and Martin (1997) observed that "different genres are different ways of using language to achieve different culturally established tasks" (p. 236). As suggested here, then, genres are *functionally* identified segments of language that are defined in terms of their social purpose.

When analyzing genres, SFL scholars divide texts into what they call *stages* of unfolding. According to van Leeuwen (1993), *stages* are sequences of speech acts that cluster together. For example, each SARS case report performs a sequence of speech acts, such as "stating the overall epidemic situation," "reporting the number of cases in SARS-infected and uninfected provinces," and so on, one after another in a sequences of stages of unfolding.

The analysis of generic structure in terms of stages is significant because both the type of information presented and the sequence in which it is revealed can have consequences for how the discourse is interpreted ideologically. However, to relate it to the ideology that underlies it we need to examine the *change* of stages in the generic structure as they unfolded over the course of the 30 case reports. For that purpose, the present study investigates the way in which the News Office included and excluded SARS case information by examining changes in generic structure of the 30 SARS case reports. Four steps are needed in this generic structure analysis: (a) the case reports are divided into chunks according to their component speech act clusters; (b) stages are differentiated and identified according to the presence of an initial and/or final speech act or a shift in the pattern of combination; (c) the nature of the change of stages in the generic structure is determined, and (d) an analysis of the change is made in relation to the anti-SARS ideology that underlies it.

Description of the data

The News Office of the Health Ministry provided a diagram (see Appendix I) that indicated the numbers of SARS cases that had been reported from different provinces, municipal cities and autonomous regions each day. This study draws on thirty reported diagrams dating from 21 April to 20 May, the month during which SARS cases underwent a full cycle from sudden rising to slow falling. The items included are about the same during the reporting period, including the diagnosed cases and the suspected cases. Within the diagnosed cases are further reported the number of patients (including medical staff), the number cured and the number dead, each with the daily totals and the accumulated totals. Within the suspected cases are reported the number of newly added cases on that day, the cases released from hospital, and the total. Table 1 shows the items reported on the SARS case statistic diagram, with an English translation below.

Although the 30 diagrams are part of the corpus, of most interest for this chapter is the way in which the number of SARS cases were reported in the form of discourse. The diagram provided the public with the objective numbers of SARS cases, but the News Office also produced a dynamic series of case reports that are taken as discourses with a particular anti-SARS ideology embedded within them. The items reported in the diagrams (see Appendix I) did not change until 19 and 20 May, when the last reporting date of newly-reported diagnosed cases and suspected cases of the day was added. This item occurs only on the last two days of the corpus and does not have a direct link with the reporting discourse. Hence, this change is considered to be unimportant for the analysis.

Generic structure of the case reports

This study examines the generic structure of the SARS case reports to determine how the change of stages in the generic structure reveals the ideology expressed

Table 1. Items reported on the SARS case statistic diagram by the Office of Health Ministry (with an English translation below)

序號	省別	臨床診斷病例		其中醫務人員		出院人數		死亡人數		疑似病例		
		新增／(其中由疑似轉為臨床診斷數)	累計	新增	累計	新增	累計	新增	累計	新增	排除	合計

序號: No.
省別: Provinces/municipal cities/automatic regions
臨床診斷病例: Diagnosed cases
新增/(其中由疑似轉為臨床診斷數): Newly added cases (transferred from suspected cases)
其中醫務人員: Medical staff in diagnosed cases
出院人數: Released from hospital
死亡人數: The dead
疑似病例: Suspected cases
新增: Newly added on the day
累計: Accumulated up to the day
排除: The released
合計: Total

in the social structure. The 9 May case report (see Appendix II) is selected for a sample description of the generic structure.

As outlined above, four steps are needed in our research. In identifying *stages* of the generic structure, the first two are applied, which are (a) to divide the case report into chunks or clusters according to its social purposes or speech acts, and (b) to identify stages according to the presence of an initial and/or final speech act or a shift in the pattern of combination. In this way, we recognize that the speech acts in the case report are either to state the overall situation or to report the number of the SARS cases (see Purpose of Stages in Table 2), and respectively label these speech acts as stages of STATING and REPORTING in the generic structure. Clauses classified as "stating" (usually only the first one or two in each report) describe some aspect of the overall SARS situation while those classified as "reporting" (usually all of the rest in each report) provide a quantifiable statistic in percentage terms or as an absolute number.

The case report is thus unpacked into different stages according to the speech acts each clause or a small group of clauses (see the Clause Domain column in Table 2) performs. To make the speech act performed more evident, key linguistic realizations of the speech act are provided (see the Key Linguistic Realizations column in Table 2). For example, in the stage of STATING (Stage 1), a relational process with verb 'have' is applied, such as: [1(a)]*On May 9, 14 prov-*

Table 2. Stages in the generic structure of the May 9 case report

Stage No.	Functionally labeled stages of generic structure	Clause domain	Purpose of stages	Key linguistic realizations
1	Stating	1–2	To state the overall epidemic situation of the country on and up to the day	Relational process (*have*) describing the situation; time adjunct as marked theme
2	Reporting	3–4	To report the number of the uninfected provinces	Relational process (*be*); inanimate subject
3	Reporting	5–6	To report the situation in affected area	Relational process (*be*) describing the situation
	further-reporting 1	5	To list provinces with no more than 10 cases	*be ... within*
	further-reporting 2	6	To report provinces having no new cases for a certain period of time	constantly, have no newly diagnosed cases for ... days
4	Reporting	7	To report the newly added diagnosed cases of the day	Relational process (*be*); time adjunct as marked theme
5	Reporting	8	To report the distribution of the diagnosed cases	Relational process (with elliptical *be*); inanimate subject
6	Reporting	9–10	To report the accumulated cases up to the day	Relational process (with elliptical *be*); inanimate subject; time adjunct as marked theme
7	Reporting	11	To report the newly added suspect cases	Relational process (with elliptical *be*); time adjunct as marked theme; inanimate subject in material process
8	Reporting	12	To report the distribution of newly added suspect cases	Relational process (with elliptical *be*); connective adjunct as marked theme
9	Reporting	13	To report the released suspect cases	Time adjunct as marked theme; relational process (with elliptical *be*)
10	Reporting	14	To report the accumulated number of suspect cases	Time adjunct as marked theme; relational process (*be*)

inces and municipal cities in the mainland have atypical pneumonia case reports. In contrast, relational process with verb *'be'* or 'elliptical *be'* is applied in the stages of REPORTING. See, for example, Stage 2 (with *be*) and Stage 5 (with elliptical *be*) in Table 2. Although this information was helpful to the researcher in identifying the various discourse functions performed in each stage, no further use of the information concerning linguistic realizations is made in this chapter.

As a result of the first two steps of our generic structure analysis, ten stages are identified in the May 9 case report, as shown in Table 2.[1] The first stage (STATING) identifies the overall epidemic situation by mentioning the on-day situation in each of the 14 provinces that provided SARS case reports. The rest of the stages (REPORTING) indicates the newly added diagnosed cases of the day, and the newly added suspect cases of the day. Occasionally, further details legitimize the statements made in the REPORTING act (e.g., in Stage 3), but with most stages, the statements presented are so plain that there seems to be no need for justification or further exemplification.

Table 2 illustrates the generic structure of the May 9 case report in terms of its stages. A close examination of the stages in the generic structure of all the 30 case reports, however, reveals that the 10 stages identified in the 9 May case report do not occur in all the 30 case reports. In addition, some case reports have stages other than those identified in the 9 May example. Table 3 lists the 14 stages identified in all 30 of the case reports, whose corresponding stage number in the 9 May case report, if there, is also provided in Table 3.

An observation of Table 3 will lead to the third step of our generic structure analysis, that is, summarizing the change of stages in the generic structures of the 30 case reports. This results in Table 4, which illustrates the distribution and change of the total stages in the 30 case reports.

We can see clearly in this table that some of the stages are deleted in the subsequent case reports (e.g. Stage 8 disappears from the 26 April report and thereafter); some are added to the subsequent reports (e.g. Stage 4 is added to the reports on 3 May and thereafter). The following section will make a detailed analysis of the stage changes in relation to the anti-SARS ideology that underlies it, which fulfils the task of the fourth step of the generic structure analysis.

---

1. The presentation the generic structure of the SARS case report follows Kong (2001, pp. 480–481, 482, 483, 485, and 487) in which he examines the generic structure of five texts of network marketing.

Table 3. Total stages in the 30 SARS case reports

Stage No.	Purpose of the stage	Corresponding stage in the 9 May report
Stage 1	To state the overall epidemic situation of the country on and up to the day	Stating (Stage 1)
Stage 2	To report the number of the uninfected provinces	Reporting (Stage 2)
Stage 3	To list provinces with no more than 10 cases	Sub-Reporting 1
Stage 4	To report provinces having no new cases for a certain period of time	Sub-Reporting 2
Stage 5	To report the newly added diagnosed cases of the day	Reporting (Stage 4)
Stage 6	To report the distribution of the diagnosed cases	Reporting (Stage 5)
Stage 7	To report the accumulated cases up to the day	Reporting (Stage 6)
Stage 8	To report local accumulated cases up to the day	(No such a stage)
Stage 9	To report the newly added suspect cases	Reporting (Stage 7)
Stage 10	To report the distribution of newly added suspect cases	Reporting (Stage 8)
Stage 11	To report the released suspect cases	Reporting (Stage 9)
Stage 12	To report the accumulated number of suspect cases	Reporting (Stage 10)
Stage 13	To report the local accumulated suspect cases	(No such stage)
Stage 14	To make a comment on the current situation	(No such stage)

Anti-SARS ideology in relation to the change of stages

As shown in Table 4, the stages constantly change in the 30 case reports, with some being added to the existing generic structure, some being removed, and some being resumed after previously being removed. The change of stages in the generic structure of the 30 case reports will be examined in order to reveal how the case reports embody a particular anti-SARS ideology.

Stages added

In the first case report on 21 April, the generic structure consists of only 8 stages: reporting the newly added diagnosed cases of the day (Stage 5), reporting the distribution of the diagnosed cases (Stage 6), reporting the accumulated cases up to the day (Stage 7), reporting the local accumulated cases up to the day (Stage 8), reporting the newly added suspect cases (Stage 9), reporting the accumulated suspect cases (Stage 12), reporting the local accumulated suspect cases (Stage 13), and commenting on the current situation (Stage 14). However, from 26 April, Stage 1, Stage 2 and Stage 10 were added to the on-day and following case reports. The content of the three new stages that appeared on the 26 April case report is as follows.

Table 4. istribution and change of stages in the 30 SARS case reports

Stage → Report on ↓	1	2	3	4	5	6	7	8	9	10	11	12	13	14
20 May*	✓	✓	✓	✓	✓	✓	✓		✓	✓	✓	✓		✓
19 May	✓	✓	✓	✓	✓	✓	✓		✓	✓	✓	✓		
18 May	✓	✓	✓	✓	✓	✓	✓		✓	✓	✓	✓		
17 May	✓	✓	✓	✓	✓	✓	✓		✓	✓	✓	✓		
16 May	✓	✓	✓	✓	✓	✓	✓		✓	✓	✓	✓		
15 May	✓	✓	✓	✓	✓	✓	✓		✓	✓	✓	✓		
14 May	✓	✓	✓	✓	✓	✓	✓		✓	✓	✓	✓		
13 May	✓	✓	✓	✓	✓	✓	✓		✓	✓	✓	✓		
12 May	✓	✓	✓	✓	✓	✓	✓		✓	✓	✓	✓		
11 May	✓	✓	✓	✓	✓	✓	✓		✓	✓	✓	✓		
10 May	✓	✓	✓	✓	✓	✓	✓		✓	✓	✓	✓		
9 May***	✓	✓	✓	✓	✓	✓	✓		✓	✓	✓	✓		
8 May	✓	✓		✓	✓	✓	✓		✓	✓	✓	✓		
7 May	✓	✓		✓	✓	✓	✓		✓	✓	✓	✓		
6 May	✓	✓		✓	✓	✓	✓		✓	✓	✓	✓		
5 May	✓	✓		✓	✓	✓	✓		✓	✓	✓	✓		
4 May	✓	✓		✓	✓	✓	✓		✓	✓	✓	✓		
3 May***	✓	✓		✓	✓	✓	✓		✓	✓	✓	✓		
2 May	✓	✓			✓	✓	✓		✓	✓	✓	✓		
1 May***	✓	✓			✓	✓	✓		✓	✓	✓	✓		
30 April	✓	✓			✓	✓	✓		✓	✓		✓		
29 April	✓	✓			✓	✓	✓		✓	✓		✓		
28 April	✓	✓			✓	✓	✓		✓	✓		✓		
27 April	✓	✓			✓	✓	✓		✓	✓		✓		
26 April**	✓	✓			✓	✓	✓		✓	✓		✓		
25 April					✓	✓	✓	✓	✓			✓	✓	
24 April					✓	✓	✓	✓	✓			✓	✓	
23 April					✓	✓	✓	✓	✓			✓	✓	
22 April					✓	✓	✓	✓	✓			✓	✓	
21 April*					✓	✓	✓	✓	✓			✓	✓	✓

***   Dates on which stages were added to the on-day reports.
**   Date on which stages were both added to and cut off from the on-day reports.
*   Dates on which the stage of comment appeared.

Stage 1   On April 26, 10 provinces and municipal cities reported newly diagnosed atypical pneumonia cases and 6 reported new suspected cases. The remaining 15 provinces report zero cases.

Stage 2   To 10:00 am on 26 April, 26 provinces and municipal cities have reported SARS cases.

Stage 10   Of the suspected cases, 173 were in Beijing, 27 in Tianjin, 9 in Hebei, 18 in Shanxi, 18 in Inner Mongolia, 1 in Heilongjiang, 4 in Shanghai, each in Zhejiang, Anhui and Henan, 3 in Hubei, 61 in Guangdong, 2 in Guangxi, 3 in Sichuan and 4 in Shan'xi.

The speech acts these three added stages perform were, respectively, to state the overall epidemic situation of the country (Stage 1), to report the number of the infected provinces (Stage 2), and to report the newly added suspect cases in different provinces (Stage 10).

Two more stages were added soon after. From 1 May, the News Office began to report the total number of released suspect cases of the day (Stage 11), and from May 3, it began to document the provinces that had no new cases for a certain period (Stage 4).

Stage 11   From 10:00 am on 30 April to 10:00 am on 1 May, 116 suspect atypical pneumonia cases were reported to have been released in various parts of mainland China. (1 May)

Stage 4   Fujian had no newly-reported cases for 25 continuous days; and Jiangxi and Shandong had no newly-reported cases for 9 days. (3 May)

While more provinces are added to the list of those that had released-suspect cases and had no new cases for a certain period, the stages by no means remained unchanging. On 9 May, another stage that reported the provinces where the total accumulated diagnosed cases were less than 10 and 5 (Stage 3) was added to the case reports.

Stage 3   Of the provinces and municipal cities where SARS was reported, Heilongjiang had no diagnosed cases; in Anhui, Shanghai, Hubei, Hunan, Gansu, Ningxia the accumulated diagnosed cases were less than 10; in Jiangsu, Zhejiang, Chongqing, Fujian, Liaoning, Jiangxi and Shandong the diagnosed cases were less than 5. (9 May)

In sum, new stages were added to the existing generic structure on four days. On 26 April, three stages were added, and on 1, 3 and 9 May one each was added. These six added stages – 1, 2, 10, 11, 4 and 3 – involved information that fitted the Ministry's beliefs and desires. For instance, with Stage 1 added, it was reported on 26 April that 10 provinces/cities reported newly-added diagnosed cases, 6 reported newly-added suspected cases, and the remaining 15 reported no cases. The Ministry may well have hoped to be seen as providing the public with detailed information, especially in the early phases of the anti-SARS social practice when there were complaints about massively inaccurate case reports.

The News Office hoped that the situation would develop in favor of the interests of its group, and its desires and beliefs found a means of expression in the added stages. On 1 May, for example, the released-suspect cases were reported. In a situation where the diagnosed and suspect cases were increasing daily, the reporting of released cases, even if the releases were of only the suspected cases, undoubtedly lifted the burden on people's minds. Such a desire became more evident when Stages 4 and 3 were added on 3 May and 9 May respectively. By reporting provinces that had no new cases for a certain period and those that had less than 5 or 10 cases reported, the Ministry was obviously attempting to reduce people's anxiety. Take Stage 4 as an illustration. It included the fact that Fujian province had no newly-reported cases for 25 continuous days. To report this on the 25th day rather than on any other of the previous days certainly reveals some of the thought processes of the News Office. The Ministry strongly desired that the reduction of people's anxiety would increase their confidence in the government.

As is frequently the case, the ideology is largely expressed in an implicit way. For example, although the addition of Stage 2 on 26 April indicates the 26 provinces and municipal cities reported SARS cases, it may also be reasonable for the News Office to imply that the rest of the provinces had not found SARS cases. This oblique way of expressing one's proposition constitutes the ambiguities of the Chinese language which, according to Hodge and Louie (1998), "are a necessary part of the ideological formation of the Chinese consciousness" and "have been used by the elite ruling group as a means to social control" (p. 99). When the SARS epidemic was at a very serious stage, to explicitly emphasize provinces where there were no SARS cases was certainly unappealing. The News Office therefore took a different approach. By adding Stage 2, which reported the number of uninfected provinces, the News Office intended to call the public's attention to the fact that some provinces had not reported SARS cases, as the total number of the provinces is a household number. This intention soon became explicit in the 3 May case report, where it is added in this particular stage that Hainan, Guizhou, Yunnan, Tibet and Qinghai had not found SARS cases.

Stages cut off

While some stages were added, other stages were cut off from the daily case reports. For example, on 26 April the details about the number of diagnosed cases (including the number of infected doctors and nurses, the released cases and the dead) in each of the infected provinces/cities (Stage 8) was removed. On the same day, Stage 13, which had reported the local accumulated suspect cases, was also removed. The content of the two stages that appeared in the 21 April case report is as follows.

Stage 8   In terms of the accumulated numbers, Guangdong had 1317 cases (including 329 medical staff), with 1136 cured and 48 dead; Beijing had 482 cases (including 78 medical staff), with 43 cured and 25 dead; Shanxi had 120 cases (including 45 medical staff), with 6 cured and 7 dead; Sichuan had 8 cases with 3 cured and 2 dead; Jiling had 3 cases; Shan'xi had 1 case; Liaoning had 2 cases; Guangxi had 14 cases, with 8 cured and 3 dead; Hunan had 6 cases, with 5 cured and 1 dead; Henan had 3 cases; Inner Mongolia had 30 cases (including 4 medical staff), with 6 dead; and Shanghai had 2 cases (21 April).

Stage 13   In terms of the accumulated number of suspect cases, Beijing had 610 cases, Shanxi had 61 cases, Guangxi had 1 case, Inner Mongolia had 48 cases, Hunan had 1 case, Sichuan had 7 cases , Shanghai had 8 cases, Henan had 1 case, Jilin had 1 case, Hebei had 7 cases, Shan'xi had 4 cases, Tianjin had 2 cases, Xinjiang had 1 case, and Chongqing had 1 case (April 21).

Removing the two stages served to distract from the serious situation in various regions. It tended to satisfy people's intuitive need to see and hear less bad news. They may intuitively have conceived that the situation was becoming less serious, and this illusion, possibly brought about by the omission of the two stages, certainly brought great comfort to the public.

The Ministry is in a dominant position in the anti-SARS social practice, and it controls access to context and discourse. The practice of removing the two stages from the discourse, as well as that of adding stages to the discourse, is a strategy that the News Office adopts to express its particular anti-SARS ideology. During the SARS epidemic it could easily block the dissemination of information that was inconsistent with its interests. By removing the two stages, the Ministry discursively exerted its influence on anti-SARS social practice.

Stage resumed

It may be a coincidence that the comment stage (Stage 14) appeared on the two ends of the continuum of the 30 SARS case reports. On the first day when the case reporting was published, a comment explained why the suspect cases in Beijing had suddenly increased. This stage of commenting did not appear again until the last case report (20 May) in our data, when a comment was made that the newly reported cases were steadily decreasing on the whole and that this should be consolidated through persistent efforts. The following is the content of this stage on 21 April and 20 May.

> Stage 14   The large increase in the reported suspected cases in Beijing was mainly the result of strict anti-SARS measures that emphasized a centralized treatment of the formerly scattered patients. (21 April)
> As seen from the local SARS reports, the newly-reported atypical pneumonia cases were steadily decreasing on the whole, but the anti-SARS task was still difficult. Persistent efforts were needed to consolidate and further the achievements. (20 May)

From the perspective of the ideological workings of the discourse, these two comments are important. The first comment may have served to calm the anxiety and complaints of the citizens of Beijing, and the second comment may have signaled a victory over the SARS epidemic. In this way, the resumed stage was ideologically manipulated so that it directed the development of anti-SARS social practice.

Social cognition and the change of stages

In the above analysis of stage changes, it is clear that an ideology was working as an underlying principle. Additions and omissions were dependent on a certain kind of mental framework in the social structure: that is, an anti-SARS ideology. In a situation where a new national leadership had just taken office, the fight against SARS was a battle that had to be won before moving on to other commitments. The shorter time the fight took, the less loss the country would suffer.

In relation to this overall situation, the News Office of the Health Ministry, when representing the case numbers in a discourse form, successfully embodied its anti-SARS ideology in the presentation of the SARS cases. In terms of access to context, the News Office decided when and how to publish the SARS discourse. For example, it decided on a wide circulation through which the SARS discourses were made public. It also decided on the daily publication for the case reporting discourse. In terms of access to discourse, the effect of this exercise of power was the most obvious. The News Office decided on the inclusion and exclusion of certain stages and thus made use of a change of stages in the generic structure of the SARS discourse.

In the representation of the case numbers by way of changing the discourse structure, then, the News Office attached more prominence to the information that went with the interests and beliefs of the Health Ministry and downgraded the information that was inconsistent with such an aim. Put another way, the preference for and ignoring of certain information in the process of discourse re-production results in the constant changing of discourse structures. In this sense, the control of access to the context and discourse produced by the News Office mediates between the discourse structure that it produced and the anti-SARS ide-ology that resulted from the social structure.

Conclusion

This study has examined 30 SARS case reports produced between 21 April and 20 May in terms of stage changes in their evolving generic structure, and has related the addition and omission of certain stages in the generic structure of the case reports to the implicit ideology that the News Office intended to produce in the fight against SARS. The News Office constantly added stages to the existing case reports that supported its interests and removed stages that were contrary to its interests. In doing so, the News Office manipulated the reporting of the number of SARS cases and thereby produced dynamic discourses that worked to inter-vene in anti-SARS social practice.

This finding becomes more convincing when other analyses of anti-SARS practice are considered. For example, Jin (2003), an analyst from the National Anti-SARS Group, produced a focused analysis of Beijing's SARS trend. Jin be-lieved that the situation in Beijing represented that of the whole country because the number of SARS cases in Beijing was 62.3%–78% of the total number of cases. According to Jin, Beijing's SARS trend was divided into three phases: from 21 to 31 April, from 1 May until 9 May and from 18 May onwards. Jin's three phases cover almost the whole period considered in this study, and the starting/end-ing dates of the three phases are strongly supported by evidence in on-day case reports. Take Jin's second phase for example. It starts at the beginning of May; in the SARS discourse data on 1 and 3 May the News Office added Stages 11 and 4 to the day's case reports. Stage 11 reported the released-suspect cases of the day and Stage 4 provided information about provinces that had no new cases for a certain period. Neither of the facts revealed by these two pieces of information had come into being on those two days, but that the News Office reported them on the two days signals an evaluation and expectation of the situation. In addition, on May 9, the end date of the second phase and starting date of the third phase, Stage 3, which reported the provinces in which there were less than 5 or 10 SARS cases, was added to the existing generic structure. Obviously, this information was con-sistent with the interests of the News Office and the Ministry. The government hoped that its measures would take effect, and this desire was conveyed to the public by the case-reporting discourse. The three phases of the anti-SARS social practice can be seen dialectically as an effect of the anti-SARS ideology embodied in manipulation of the case reports.

The significance of this study lies, then, primarily in the textual analysis of the *set* of SARS case report that reveals the anti-SARS ideology of the News Office. A single case report may be considered as establishing a genre and thus as a form of participating in social practice. Seen separately, the single report remains as objective as the case numbers do in the statistical diagram, but seen in succession with one another, the 30 case reports embody the anti-SARS ideology. As is analyzed in the present study, the constant change of stages in the 30 case reports is a way of representing the anti-SARS social practice of China's Ministry of Health.

References

Eggins, S., & Martin, J. (1997). Genres and registers of discourse. In T. A. van Dijk (Ed.), *Discourse as structure and process* (pp. 230–256). London: Sage.

Fairclough, N. (1985). Critical and descriptive goals in discourse analysis. *Journal of Pragmatics, 9,* 737–763.

Fairclough, N. (2000). Discourse, social theory and social research: The discourse of welfare reform. *Journal of Sociolinguistics, 4*(2), 163–195.

Fairclough, N. (2001). The discourse of new labour: Critical discourse analysis. In M. Wetherell, S. Taylor, & S. Yates (Eds.), *Discourse as data* (pp. 229–266). London: Sage, in Association with the Open University.

Fairclough, N. (2003). *Analysing discourse: Textual analysis for social research.* London and New York: Routledge.

Hodge, B., & Louie, K. (1998). *The politics of Chinese language and culture.* London and New York: Routledge.

Jin, S. (2003, May 18). http://www.sina.com.cn. Xinhua.

Kong, K. C. C. (2001). Marketing of belief: Intertextual construction of network marketer's identity. *Discourse & Society, 12*(4), 473–503.

Van Dijk, T. A. (1993). Principles of critical discourse analysis. In M. Toolan (Ed.), *Critical discourse analysis: Critical concepts in linguistics* (four volumes), vol. II (pp. 104–141). London and New York: Routledge.

Van Dijk, T. A. (1995). Discourse semantics and ideology. *Discourse & Society, 6*(2), 243–289.

Van Dijk, T. A. (1998). Opinions and ideologies in the press. In A. Bell & P. Garrett (Eds.), *Approaches to media discourse* (pp. 21–63). Oxford: Blackwell.

Van Dijk, T. A. (1999). Discourse analysis as ideology analysis. In C. Schäffner & A. L. Wenden (Eds.), *Language and peace* (pp. 17–33). Amsterdam: Harwood Academic Publishers.

Van Leeuwen, T. (1993). Genre and field in critical discourse analysis: A synopsis. *Discourse & Society, 4*(2), 193–223.

Wodak, R. (2001). What CDA is about – A summary of its history, important concepts and its developments. In R. Wodak & M. Meyer (Eds.), *Methods of critical discourse analysis* (pp. 1–13). London: Sage.

Appendix I: Diagram of the numbers of SARS cases reported on May 9

全國內地非典型肺炎疫情統計表（截至5月9日10時）

序號	省別	臨床診斷病例 新增／（其中由疑似轉為臨床診斷數）	累計	其中醫務人員 新增	累計	出院人數 新增	累計	死亡人數 新增	累計	疑似病例 新增	排除	合計
1	北京	48(28)	2177[1]	3	372	16	168	2	114	54	87	1425
2	天津	9(5)	141	2	66	0	2	1	6	11	1	123
3	河北	9(4)	156	0	15	2	11	2	8	6	3	109
4	山西	11(6)	400[2]	0	76	15	69	0	17	14	22	138
5	內蒙古	20(10)	284[3]	3	42	3	16	1	17	10	5	193
6	遼寧	0	2	0	0	0	0	0	0	0	0	3
7	吉林	0	26	0	6	0	0	0	3	0	0	7
8	黑龍江	0	0	0	0	0	0	0	0	0	0	4
9	上海	0	6	0	0	0	0	0	1	4	4	12
10	江蘇	0	5	0	0	0	0	0	0	1	0	23
11	浙江	0	4	0	0	0	0	0	0	0	1	4
12	安徽	0	9	0	0	0	0	0	2	0	13
13	福建	0	3	0	0	1	3	0	0	0	0	1
14	江西	0	1	0	0	0	0	0	0	0	2
15	山東	0	1	0	0	0	0	0	0	1	1	1
16	河南	0	15	0	1	1	3	0	0	0	14
17	湖北	0	6	0	1	0	0	0	0	1	15
18	湖南	0	6	0	0	0	5	0	1	0	3
19	廣東	17(7)	1502	1	345	15	1288	0	56	38	36	414
20	廣西	0	20	0	0	0	9	0	3	0	1	3
21	重慶	0	3	0	0	0	0	0	0	0	7
22	四川	2(2)	13	0	0	0	4	0	2	1	0	17
23	陝西	1	12	0	1	0	2	0	0	1	1	27
24	甘肅	1	7	0	0	0	0	0	1	0	3
25	寧夏	0	6	0	0	0	2	0	1	0	2	5
合計		118(62)	4805	9	925	53	1582	6	230	144	164	2566

[1] 北京排除原臨床診斷病例7例（其中醫務人員1例，轉疑似病例2例）。

[2] 山西排除原臨床診斷病例2例。

[3] 內蒙古排除原臨床診斷病例2例。

Appendix II: The 9 May SARS case report with its English translation (clauses are marked out)

[1(a)]On May 9, 14 provinces and municipal cities in the mainland have atypical pneumonia case reports, [(b)]including 8 that report new diagnosed and suspect cases, 1 new diagnosed case and 5 new suspected cases. [2(a)]The remaining 17 provinces report no new cases. [3(a)]To 10:00 am of May 9, provinces and municipal cities [(b)]that have reported SARS cases are 25. [4(a)]Six provinces, Hainan, Guizhou, Yunnan, Tibet, Qinghai and Xinjiang have not reported SARS cases. [5(a)]In the provinces and municipal cities [(b)]that have reported the epidemic, Heilongjiang has no diagnosed cases; [(c)]in provinces such as Anhui, Shanghai, Hubei, Hunan, Gansu, Ningxia, etc., the accumulated diagnosed cases are less than 10; [(d)]in provinces such as Jiangsu, Zhejiang, Chongqing, Fujian, Liaoning, Jiangxi and Shandong, etc., the diagnosed cases are less than 5. [6(a)]Fujian has had no new cases for 31 days on end, [(b)]Hunan has had no new diagnosed cases for 18 days on end, [(c)]Shandong has had no new diagnosed cases for 15 days on end, [(d)]Guangxi has had no new diagnosed cases for 7 days on end, [(e)]Niangxia has had no new diagnosed cases for 6 days on end and [(f)]Jiangxi has had no new diagnosed cases for 5 days on end.

[7(a)]From 10:00 am of May 8 to 10:00 am of May 9, various parts of mainland China reported 118 diagnosed atypical pneumonia cases [(b)]including 62 cases that were transferred from suspect cases), [(c)]53 cases cured and released from hospital and [(d)] 6 cases of death. [8(a)]Among the diagnosed cases, 48 are in Beijing [(b)]28 are cases transferred from suspect cases and [(c)]20 are new cases), [(d)]16 are cured [(e)]and 2 are dead; [(f)]9 are in Tianjin [(g)]5 are cases transferred from suspect cases), [(h)]and 1 is dead; [(i)]9 are in Hebei [(j)]4 are cases transferred from suspect cases, [(k)]and 2 are cured [(l)]and 2 are the dead; [(m)]11 are in Shanxi, [(n)]6 are cases transferred from suspect cases and [(o)]15 are cured; [(p)]20 are in Inner Mongolia,[(q)](10 are cases transferred from suspect cases), [(r)]3 are cured and [(s)]one is dead; [(t)]one is cured in Fujia; [(u)]one is cured in Henan; [(v)]17 cases are in Guangdong; [(w)]7 are cases transferred from suspect cases and [(x)]15 are the cured); [(y)]2 are in Sichua [(z)]which are transferred from suspect cases; [(aa)]one case is in Shan'xi; and [(ab)]one case is in Gansu. [9(a)] To 10:00 am of May 9, an accumulated number of 4805 atypical pneumonia cases have been reported in various parts of mainland China [(b)]925 are medical staff), [(c)]the accumulated cured and released from hospital are 1582 [(d)]and the dead are 230. [10(a)]Those [(b)]who are now receiving treatment in hospital are 2993. [11(a)]From10:00am of May 8 to 10:00am of May 9, various parts report [(b)]that the newly emerged atypical pneumonia suspect cases are 144. [12(a)] Among these are 54 in Beijing, [(b)]11 in Tianjin; [(c)]6 in Hebei; [(d)]14 in Shanxi; [(e)]10 in Inner Mogolia; [(f)]4 in Shanghai [(g)]one in Jiangsu; [(h)]2 in Anhui; [(i)] 1 each in Shangdong and Hubei; [(j)]38 in Guangdong; and [(k)]1 each in Sichuan and Shan'xi.

[13(a)]From 10:00 am of May 8 to 10:00 am of May 9, various provinces of mainland China also reported 164 released suspect atypical pneumonia cases, [(b)]among which 87 are in Beijing, [(c)]36 are in Guangdong, [(d)]22 are in Shanxi, [(e)]5 are in Inner Mongolia, [(f)]4 are in Shanghai, [(g)]3 are in Hebei, [(h)]2 are in Ningxia and [(i)]one in Tianjin, Zhejiang, Shangdong, Guangxi, Shan'xi each. [14(a)]To 10:00 am of May 9, the accumulated number of suspect atypical pneumonia cases is 2566.

PART III

Constructions of SARS in Singapore and Taiwan

CHAPTER 8

"Triumph over adversity"

Singapore mobilizes Confucian values to combat SARS

Ian Weber, Tan Howe Yang and Law Loo Shien
Texas A&M University / Nanyang Technological University

This chapter explores how the Singapore government worked hand-in-hand with the media to draw the nation together under the banner of a modified and popularized version of Confucianism during the SARS crisis in 2003. Specifically, it focuses on the ways governmental leaders used civic discourse to renegotiate citizenship through the media's discursive practices in order to gain public compliance with government directives. Employing Gee's (2002) discourse analysis framework, this study examines reports published by Singapore's flagship newspaper, the *Straits Times*, to discover the relevant discursive themes that link into and perpetuate the national mythology of "triumph over adversity." The study found that communication strategies contributed significantly to the enrichment of a self-sustaining mythology that symbolically ties citizens to national goals. By demonstrating how socially responsible citizens can contribute directly to the nation, the mythology helped Singaporeans to identify with national strength and character exemplified by the heroism of the medical community during the SARS crisis. Adding successful management of the SARS crisis to Singapore's mythic lore of "triumph over adversity" should reinforce the government's efforts to motivate citizens to be socially responsible whenever the next crisis challenges Singapore's national character.

Introduction

SARS became a major international challenge for many governments in the first six months of 2003 when the disease spread from the southern Chinese province of Guangdong to 28 countries, including Hong Kong, Taiwan, Vietnam, Canada, and Singapore. According to the World Health Organization (WHO), a total of 8,437 cases were confirmed with 813 fatalities, including 33 deaths in Singapore (Chua, 2004). Many countries felt the economic effects of SARS, with travel limitations placed on all affected countries. For example, Singapore's tourism industry experienced its first ever quarterly loss of S$312 million by its national carrier Singapore Airlines (Sim 2003; From bullock carts, 2004; Sreenvasan 2004; Chua 2004). Furthermore, the retail industry was adversely affected as the fear of infection gripped Singaporeans, forcing them to stay indoors. Accordingly, Singapore's Gross Domestic Product (GDP) was reduced by between 0.5 and 2.5% (Singapore's rapid response, 2003). Responding to the outbreak, Singapore Deputy Prime Minister Lee Hsien Loong[1] (2003) labeled SARS a "national crisis" with "catastrophic consequences" in a parliamentary speech in April 2003.

In spite of its serious losses, Singapore is recognized internationally as having successfully managed the outbreak of SARS. Government efforts garnered praise from the WHO as a "model" of crisis management for other nations to emulate (Henson 2003). The Singapore government enforced strict measures to contain the outbreak, including Home Quarantine Orders, contact tracing, provision of thermometers to all residents, and implementation of revolutionary thermal imaging scanners at immigration checkpoints.[2] However, it was the Singapore government's policy of open communication, which mobilized its population to help contain the SARS epidemic, that set the city-state apart from other affected areas such as China, Taiwan, and Hong Kong (World Bank commends, 2003; Chua 2004, p. 182).

This chapter examines how the Singapore government and the media worked hand-in-hand to draw the nation together under the banner of a modified and popularized Confucianism during this time of national crisis. The study extends Kluver and Weber's (2003) work on the ways in which governmental leaders use civic discourse to renegotiate citizenship by examining the discursive practices employed by the media to gain public compliance with government directives

---

1.   Lee Hsien Loong was appointed Prime Minister of Singapore in August 2004, replacing Goh Chok Tong who stepped down from the position after 14 years in power, including overseeing Singapore's response to the SARS crisis. Goh was appointed Senior Minister, second in rank only to the Prime Minister.

2.   Thermal imaging scanners continue to be used extensively at airports in Hong Kong, China, Taiwan, and Singapore.

during the SARS crisis. Employing Gee's (2002) discourse analysis framework, this chapter examines articles published by Singapore's flagship daily newspaper the *Straits Times* during the SARS crisis to explore the discursive themes that link into, and perpetuate, the national mythology of "triumph over adversity."

National identity, Confucianism, and the media

On May 30, 2003, the WHO removed Singapore from its list of SARS-affected countries, and thanked the nation for its excellent collaboration in the previous months (Chang 2003). The government's vindication by the WHO acknowledged that the SARS outbreak was effectively contained, with the economy returning to pre-crisis levels.[3] Singapore's success in containing the virus led Prime Minister Goh Chok Tong to praise Singaporeans in his 2003 National Day Rally Speech:

> A crisis reveals the true character of a people. Singaporeans passed the SARS test with distinction. We were at war with SARS. To overcome the enemy, we knew we had to work together as a nation. And we did. We closed ranks and stood with each other. We helped each other without regard for race, religion, or social position. During this crisis, I saw a national spirit I have never seen before. Our country bonded with stout hearts, tenacity and determination. SARS did not break Singapore. It made us stronger. I am very proud of our solidarity.   (Goh 2003a)

Goh's speech articulates the type of civic discourse that constitutes the grander narrative of "triumph over adversity," which encapsulates how Singapore has attempted to shape its national identity during its short 40-year history. However, before the SARS crisis doubts were cast upon the effectiveness of such discourse. For example, Kluver and Weber (2003) argued that the persuasiveness of such discourse had been blunted by the effects of rapid globalization, which "undermined a consciousness of shared identity and shared opportunities" among Singaporeans, resulting in a failure to generate an effective "self-sustaining national mythology" that would "tie its citizens to its shores" (p. 384). Utilizing Barthes (1972) notion of national mythologies[4] and grounding their analysis in the memoirs of

---

3. In spite of Singapore's success, SARS continued to be a major concern, with a second, smaller outbreak occurring in China in 2004. Accordingly, the disease continues to be an issue epidemiologically, as well as politically and socially, for countries with close contact with China through business, travel, and tourism.

4. A central point to these discussions on mythology concerns the way certain images and symbols are negotiated to reinterpret national identity through the national myth or, in Barthes' (1972) terms, the space "between reality and man, between description and explanation, be-

Singapore's founding Prime Minister, Lee Kuan Yew (2000), as well as speeches from top governmental leaders and citizen participation in national debates, Kluver and Weber (2003) argued that Singapore's political leadership had created a "national myth" of economic survival from several national crises since independence in 1965 as a way of tying Singaporeans to a common theme of economic resilience through adversity.

In light of Singapore's success in mobilizing its citizens into a cohesive nation acting as "one people" to fight against SARS, it is timely to re-examine Kluver and Weber's (2003) analysis of an ineffectual "self-sustaining national mythology" designed to combat national crises. Past studies on Singapore's national identity show how the government has attempted to engender a strong sense of belonging among Singaporeans since 1965 (Chua & Kuo 1995). At the heart of these mobilizing processes is the control exerted over Singaporeans by "a coherent elite" made up of the judiciary, paramilitary, commerce, and public bureaucracy, as well as by academic and media institutions (Ho 2000, p. 94). From its position of power, the Singaporean government has propagated through various political discourses social ideals and values that were deemed central to the continued prosperity of the city-state. Highly pragmatic, the government used the discourse of "triumph over adversity" as "a rallying cry" for Singaporeans and as a justification for government policies to overcome crises such as riots (1960s), oil shortage (1970s), economic downturns (1980s and 1990s) (Mauzy & Milner 2002), and negative aspects of westernization (Kluver & Weber 2003). The common thread within each of these public communication campaigns was the proliferation of a government-defined set of "Asian values," which was thought to provide the social glue to maintain the political and social stability of the country during times of crisis.

At the core of the broadly defined "Asian values" framework were the government's attempts to "entrench an elaborate Confucian philosophy in the ideological landscape of Singapore" (Chua 1998). For example, in 1982, the government introduced Confucian ethics'[5] classes into Singapore's education system. This was

---

tween object and knowledge" (p. 159). This plays out in the Singapore context in the relationship between national identity, global-local dynamic, and the process of myth-making, which helps to inform and frame Singapore's renegotiation of citizenship (Kluver & Weber 2003, p. 373).

5.   Confucianism encapsulates both social and political philosophy. Confucius' social philosophy largely revolves around the concept of *ren*, "compassion" or "loving others." Practicing such concern for others involved deprecating oneself. While ritual forms often have to do with the more narrow relations of family and clan, *ren* is to be practised broadly and informs one's interactions with all people. Confucius warned those in power that they should not oppress or take for granted even the lowliest of their subjects. He regarded devotion to parents and older siblings as the most basic form of promoting the interests of others before one's own and teaches

followed by the engagement of eight overseas Chinese scholars who gave public lectures, conducted seminars, and held meetings with government ministers to conceptualize Confucian doctrines relevant to Singapore. The Institute of East Asian Philosophy was established a year later to promote the study of philosophies, specifically Confucianism. Kuo (1996) suggests that "Confucian ethics was being promoted at a societal level . . . following a format similar to those of numerous other campaigns in Singapore" (p. 295).

Governmental efforts to promote Confucian thinking, however, were poorly subscribed by the public (Chua 1998). The English-educated Chinese disapproved, viewing the strategy as a conspiracy to legitimize authoritarian government. Non-Chinese viewed the move as another way to increase Chinese dominance in Singapore,[6] while few students attended Confucian ethics' classes. Brown (1993) argues that public debate and resistance to the government's initiative to impose a Confucian-based value system on Singaporeans exposed the weakness and ambiguity of Singapore's national identity. Accordingly, Confucian ethics classes were phased out in 1990. However, as Tu (1996) argues, the Confucian movement had already realized its aim of sensitizing Singaporean Chinese to the positive values of the country's Confucian heritage, laying the foundation for the gradual and subtle introduction of a modified and popularized version in subsequent years.

Following the unsuccessful Confucian movement in the 1980s, the Singapore government revised its thinking on the adopted "Asian values" framework and proposed a White Paper outlining a framework of "Five Shared Values", as a national ideology to provide grounding for Singaporeans to face future challenges. Singapore's "Five Shared Values" include: a) nation before community and society above self; b) family as the basic unit of society; c) community support and respect for the individual; d) consensus not conflict; and e) racial and religious harmony. While the "Five Shared Values" framework was fully compatible with Confucianism, a presidential report on the White Paper insisted that the government never intended to allow the SHARED VALUES to become "a subterfuge for imposing

---

that only those who have learned self-discipline can accomplish such altruism. Learning self-restraint involves studying and mastering *li*, the ritual forms and rules of propriety through which one expresses respect for superiors and enacts his [sic] role in society in such a way that he himself [sic] is worthy of respect and admiration. A concern for propriety should inform everything that one says and does. For Confucius, what characterized superior rulership was the possession of *de* or "virtue." Conceived of as a kind of moral power that allows one to win a following without recourse to physical force, such "virtue" also enabled the ruler to maintain good order in his state without troubling himself [sic] and by relying on loyal and effective deputies (Riegel 2002).

6.   Singapore consists of four ethnic groups, of which the Chinese dominate with over three-quarters (76.7%) of the total population of 4 million people.

Chinese Confucian values" on non-Chinese Singaporeans. The report indicated the relevance of Confucian values to Singapore, but acknowledged that it would also have to be "brought up to date and reconciled with other ideas which are also essential parts of our ethos" (Kuo 1996, p. 297).

Although little academic research has been conducted on the success of such programs, Chua and Kuo (1995) argue that the "Five Shared Values" framework remains "a floating signifier" for Singaporeans because it is neither enshrined in the Constitution nor an actionable piece of legislation. However, the government has managed to build the validity of this values framework using its close relationship to the Singapore media. As Bokhorst-Heng (2002) suggests, the centrality of the national agenda and nation building to the role of the media in Singapore "is unambiguous in the many speeches government leaders have given on the topic. It is made clear both by framing the role of the media against what is *not* and by defining what it *is*" (pp. 559–560). This role was reinforced by the then Deputy Prime Minister Lee following the SARS crisis, suggesting the local media was vital to "building a civic society," by "playing a constructive role in nation building" (Chua 2004). The close alignment of the media with the political agenda of nation building is a result of the complex interaction between direct legislation to control local and foreign media licensing and content, and the informal relationships between government officials and editors of the local press and broadcast media management.

Method

This chapter employs a qualitative approach to examine the discursive practices employed by the media to gain public compliance with government directives during the SARS epidemic in Singapore. It focuses specifically on the English-language daily newspaper the *Straits Times* to explore relevant discourse themes that link into, and perpetuate, the national mythology of "triumph over adversity." According to Graham (1999), it is through discourse that people negotiate their social milieu, comprised of entire networks constructed by interactions and processes. Within this network of interaction and processes, the domain of language is where social perceptions of values and power are created and mediated. Accordingly, language is what enables humans to understand, interpret, and navigate their world. Because language is so essential in human affairs, we draw on the discourse analysis framework offered by Gee (2002) to gain a deeper, richer understanding of the dominant language themes surrounding the Singapore media's handling of the SARS crisis.

The *Straits Times* was chosen as the media source to study because it has the largest distribution figures of all print media in Singapore, and is considered the most credible. Its daily circulation figures exceed 400,000 copies (*Straits Times* 2004), with a readership of more than 1.3 million people per day (ACNielsen 2004). Articles were drawn from the publication during the height of the SARS crisis (March 1, 2003) to the day after the country's definitive National Day Rally Speech on August 9, 2003. A search of newspaper databases Factiva and Lexis Nexis using the keyword "SARS" returned 1,056 articles. Each article was cross-referenced against the broader discourse themes – government, nation building and social cohesion – identified by Kluver and Weber (2003) in their analysis of Singapore's approach to forming a national identity though civic discourse. Given this approach, a purposive sample of 160 articles was defined for analysis, with two Singaporean research assistants producing a category framework comprised of three dominant themes – social responsibility, sacrifice, and government paternalism – in the pre-coding phase of the study. The coders also identified several recurring metaphors (e.g. *enemy*, *battle* and *heroes*) within the sample, which were interwoven with the dominant themes to provide persuasive traction for the Singapore media reports on SARS.

In examining the language used by the *Straits Times* to construct meaning, the study utilized a working assumption that any portion of text will be simultaneously representing, forming identities, and establishing relations (Fairclough 1995, p. 5). Within such language constructs, Gee (2002) argues that there are two ways in which meaning is attached to words and phrases in actual use: situated meaning and cultural models. *Situated meaning* refers to an image or pattern that we assemble "on the spot" as we communicate in a given context, based on our construal of that context and our past experiences (p. 80). Situated meanings, however, do not just *reside* in the individual mind; very often they are *negotiated* between people in, and through, communicative social interaction (discourse). Doing so, it is necessary to account for the meaning of such language constructs within the larger context of an ongoing relationship between Singapore's government and its citizenry for the purpose of identity construction and nation-building. As the communication, and indeed relationship, between government and citizens develops over time, participants continually revise situated meanings. For example, words such *war*, *enemy* and *heroes* can be general in meaning and also have situated meanings within different contexts because of their association with "cultural models." For Gee (2002), *cultural models* refer to "storylines," or families of connected images (like mental movies), or "informal" theories shared by people belonging to specific social or cultural groups.

When placed in the context of national stories or mythologies (see Barthes 1972; Kluver & Weber 2003), larger pieces of information have their own characteristics and high-level organizations. That is, such large bodies of information have characteristic parts (such as social responsibility, sacrifice, and paternalism), which are supported by smaller parts (words and phrases, such as *war, enemy* or *heroes*). Such large bodies of information can be equated with the cultural model, as opposed to its situated meanings. In order to see the patterning of such language that builds meaning, Gee (2002) offers a story structure of setting, catalyst, crisis, evaluation, resolution, and coda. Accordingly, the *setting* provides the scene in terms of time, space, and characters; a *catalyst* sets the problem; a *crisis* builds the problem to the point of requiring a resolution; an *evaluation* is material that makes clear why the story is interesting and worth telling; a *resolution* solves the problem set by the story; and the *coda* closes the story (p. 12). Together, Gee's (2002) approach forms a strategically competent way to undertake discourse analysis or the "reciprocal and cyclical process in which we shuttle back and forth between the structure (form and design) of a piece of language and the situated meanings it is attempting to build about the world, identities and relationships" (p. 99).

Triumph over adversity: Social responsibility, sacrifice and paternalism

The Singapore government's overarching strategy to curb the spread of SARS was to isolate and contain the virus. This strategy required the cooperation of the general public as government communication directed people to undertake behavioral and attitudinal change. For example, people were advised to check their temperatures daily, practice good personal hygiene, and obey quarantine orders dutifully should they be served with one. To gain public compliance with such directives, government officials framed communicative responses to the crisis in terms of "social responsibility" and "sacrifice," under girded by "government paternalism."

The social responsibility theme

Speeches, news reports and editorial commentaries called for Singaporeans to exercise self-restraint and cooperation during the SARS crisis, drawing on the hierarchy-based Confucian value of putting "nation before community and society above self." For example, the *Straits Times* published an open letter to the public by Prime Minister Goh highlighting the emancipatory benefits of following the rules, procedures, and recommendations. He stressed that Singapore would only overcome SARS if "everyone played their part" (Goh 2003b). Goh also emphasized the various socially responsible behaviors that people should adopt. Accordingly, the onus was placed on people to be community oriented by truthfully reporting their symptoms and history of contacts regardless of their self-interests, so that no suspected cases would go unchecked at the community level. Measures were also outlined in the press and broadcast media for people who were not socially re-sponsible, including electronically tagging of offenders who failed to comply with government quarantine directives. This focus reflects Gee's (2002) notion of estab-lishing the setting and catalyst, in which the main characters (citizens and govern-ment) and problem (life-threatening disease) were laid out for the public. This was exemplified by Prime Minister Goh (2003b) when he warned Singaporeans that:

> Once SARS spreads through the community, we risk losing control of it, and it we will not be able to isolate and contain it . . . the chain is only as strong as its weakest link, and everyone has an important part to play.   (p. 2)

To encourage the public to be socially responsible, the government adopted a range of powerful analogies in its public communication that would resonate within the Singaporean consciousness. Prominent in the discourse was the use of war-related metaphors to reinforce the struggle of good over evil. For exam-ple, government officials routinely equated this struggle against SARS as "a battle against an unknown enemy," with doctors and healthcare workers at the "front line." Prime Minister Goh, for example, accessed these war metaphors often in speeches and at press conferences, suggesting that "every Singaporean is a soldier in the fight against SARS. . . We have armed every household with a thermometer as our weapon" (Khalik 2003, p. 12). During the height of the crisis, Deputy Prime Minister Lee also framed the response to SARS as one in which "public health, economy, and society are the most critical battlefronts" (Henson 2003).

The ability to tie the SARS crisis to the notion of war links into Kuo's (1996) idea of "a floating signifier." Because of the speed with which SARS emerged, the Singapore government could not rely on law enshrined in the Constitution nor an actionable piece of legislation to gain compliance with directives from its citi-zenry. Nor could authorities implement harsh, draconian measures without eras-ing the trust that had been built up between citizenry and authorities in recent years, particularly in relation to the adoption of a more consultative governmental approach (i.e., consensus not conflict). Therefore, the government chose to link into established levels of patriotism, which had attempted to tie citizenry to the nation throughout its short history. As military analyst at the Institute of Defence and Strategic Studies, Brigadier-General (Ret.) Law Chwee Kiat suggests:

> War against SARS is a catch phrase used by the Government to describe the en-tire national effort to deal with the outbreak. It is an icon that the Government wants the general public to associate with something that threatens the existence

of the state. The virus is communicated as the enemy, a threat that has to be demolished. It is a signifier used to galvanize Singaporeans to take whatever precautions necessary.

(cited in Long 2003)

To give the "war" metaphors persuasive traction, the government "naturalized" the language by using Chinese dialects and Singlish[7] in public communication campaigns and television programs. For example, local broadcast stations Channel 8 and Channel U hosted live call-in forums to talk about SARS using a range of dialects – the first time the government had permitted such usage within the national media since 1982. Government officials also spoke in dialects in speeches and media interviews. For example, Deputy Prime Minister Lee and Senior Minister of State Khaw Boon Wan, head of the virus combat team of junior ministers, both spoke in dialect during television phone-in and forum programs and at press conferences. The temporary reversal of government policy was the result of initial media criticism that the campaigns needed to be more effectively targeted by reaching out to those people who only understood dialects.

In spite of this early criticism, Singapore's media quickly resumed its social responsibility role, as defined by its close relationship with government, to help authorities manage society and thus the national crisis. The *Straits Times* newspaper weaved implicit approval and support for the preventative measures into news and feature articles and editorial commentary on SARS. Many news headlines assumed a parochial call-to-action for Singaporeans to change their attitudes and behaviors: DRACONIAN? SINGAPORE IS JUST DOING WHAT IT NEEDS TO FIGHT SARS; DON'T PANIC OVER SARS; and LET'S GET BACK TO BUSINESS OF LIVING.

As the health crisis deepened in May 2003, television broadcast competitors Singapore Press Holdings (SPH), Media Corporation of Singapore (MediaCorp), and StarHub Cable TV joined forces to establish a dedicated SARS Channel, which transmitted from noon to midnight each day. Popular celebrities from each television group were used to promote government measures and discuss SARS related issues. Local television celebrity Phua Chu Kang, a fictitious character played by popular comedian Gurmit Singh, launched a song called the "SARvivor Rap," which was commissioned by the Singapore Health Ministry. The rap song used Singlish in the music video, with lyrics such as "Some say leh, some say lah," "Don't kak-pui [spit]all over the place" and "Don't do things and become a regretter." At the launch of the SARS channel, SPH Chief Executive Officer Alan

---

7.   Singlish is a form of language structured around a combination of English, Malay and Chinese words, phrases and grammar that emerged from grassroots Singaporeans as a cultural identifier within the city-state.

Chan suggested the media's united front was "a natural move" and "further entrenched Singapore's media industry as responsive, responsible, and willing to serve the public interest" (Media rivals team, 2003).

The sacrifice theme

An extension of the "social responsibility" theme, where every Singaporean was asked to play their part for the collective good, was the public praise of the "heroic" medical community in appreciation for their "sacrifice" in the fight against SARS. Such references to "sacrifice" began from within the medical community early in the crisis, and were subsequently carried forward by the government, media, and the public. The *Straits Times*, for example, used the government's war analogy hand-in-hand with survival stories, promoting the victims of SARS as "war heroes." News reports linked these heroes directly to the healthcare profession as a way to counter the public fear towards hospitals, doctors, and nurses as the number of deaths continued to rise. For example, a *Sunday Times* story titled "DON'T TREAT FAMILIES AND FRIENDS LIKE CRIMINALS" called on the public to praise not ostracize nurses. The story came in response to information that some Singaporeans on public transport networks had shunned nurses, and even their own families, which ran counter to the "Five Shared Values" framework where community support and respect for the individual and the family form the basic unit of Singaporean society. In so doing, the discourse attempts to build from the catalyst or problem to establish the significance of the crisis; in this situation the erosion of Singapore's foundational core values, which threatened the nation's social stability. Responding to the challenge, the *Straits Times*' "Letters to the Editor" section ran numerous comments from the public chastising such discrimination as the deeds of "ugly Singaporeans," as a way to urge citizens to support the sacrifices made by the medical profession and families in general, thus reinforcing the values of community support for the individual and consensus not conflict.

These sacrifices were acknowledged and rewarded by the government, who announced it would match public donations to *The Courage Fund* dollar-for-dollar, in addition to contributing $1 million. The Singapore Medical Association and the Singapore Nurses Association set up the Fund to garner financial support for the healthcare workers and the families of SARS patients who had suffered or fallen ill. Further public recognition was exhibited through National Day commemoration ceremony involving 4,000 Singaporeans and the awarding of medals of valor to the medical community of doctors, nurses and healthcare professionals for their "sacrifices," much like soldiers and generals who performed valiantly in combat.

Posthumous awards were also presented in honor of the "fallen" SARS victims. Prime Minister Goh identified two of Singapore's fallen "war heroes" – Dr. Alexandre Chao and nurse Madam Hamidah Ismail, who both passed away in the line of duty – to illustrate the sacrifices people had made for the nation. In identifying such sacrifices, the discourse attempts to clarify, or in Gee's (2002) terms evaluate, the situation in a way that Singaporeans could relate the battle against SARS to previous shared experiences in which the nation had successfully overcome crises. For instance, Goh (2003c) used the story of people's sacrifices during SARS to demonstrate the type of character that all Singaporeans should strive for:

> I believe Singaporeans are made of sterner stuff. I believe they have fighting spirit. . . . Take for instance our doctors, nurses and other personnel working to help SARS-infected patients. They have conducted themselves magnificently throughout the crisis. They have displayed great resolve, and a noble sense of professional responsibility. . . . This is the kind of steel in our character that will see Singapore through hard times. We should honor them.   (Goh 2003c)

The theme of "sacrifice" supported the government's overarching social responsibility discourse by imparting a sense of nobility and bravery to the public's adherence to SARS measures. Such displays of positive community values in the line of national duty were communicated as commendable and thus to be emulated by all Singaporeans when confronted with crisis. By publicly commending the sacrificial courage of Singaporeans and the medical community, the government placed a premium on the value of "community above self," a cornerstone of the "Five Shared Values" framework.

Government paternalism: Moral virtue and compassion

In addition to the strategic use of language to gain public compliance with SARS measures, other symbolic events were instrumental in persuading the public to adopt the call for "social responsibility" and to make "sacrifices" for the community and the nation. Singapore's Senior Minister Lee Kuan Yew told the media how he never left home without his thermometer. Member of Parliament, Dr. Tan Cheng Bock, imposed voluntary quarantine on himself when he found he had treated a SARS-infected patient. Prime Minister Goh also lunched with local media editors at the Rendezvous Restaurant to show Singaporeans that it was safe to be in public places. These stories illustrated to the Singapore public the "moral virtue" of a government leading by example. By showing the people that government leaders practised what they preached, the examples served to "naturalize" and "legitimize" the public discourse of "social responsibility" and "sacrifice" for all Singaporean citizens.

Linked to this notion of moral virtue (*de*) was the government's compassion (*ren*) for its citizenry, whose respect for authority was soundly tested under the growing fears that SARS might spread through the nation's school system. Many parents lobbied the government for a delay in re-opening schools after the weeklong March break through "Letters to the Editor" in the *Straits Times*. These parents argued that children who had traveled overseas during the break could have returned with SARS without exhibiting any symptoms because of the virus's 10-day incubation period. Initial response by the Singapore Ministry of Health was to advise parents to monitor their children for symptoms of SARS if they had been to Hong Kong, Guangdong, or Hanoi. The health ministry claimed the number of SARS cases then did not warrant a need to close schools, as this was not recommended by the WHO. However, three days after the schools reopened, the first child infection was recorded, followed by the deaths of two SARS patients. The education ministry then decided to assuage the fears of worried parents by going beyond the WHO recommendations and closing all schools under the tertiary level for two weeks. The move showed government compassion for the worries and concerns of parents. This action served to legitimize the government's position as a caring, paternalistic government that acts in the line with Singapore's "Five Shared Values" in relation to families as the basic unit of society and achieving a consensus (not conflict) through communicative action.

Discussion: Reaping the rewards of a Confucian foundation

In the final analysis, five factors contributed to Singapore's success: (a) single-mindedness; (b) open communication; (c) clear leadership structure, (d) cooperation from Singaporeans; and (e) courage of healthcare workers (Chua 2004, p. 182). From a leadership perspective, the Singapore government linked Confucian values of moral leadership (*de*), compassion (*ren*) and respect (*li*), to the "Five Shared Values" framework to successfully implement communication strategies that helped to contain the SARS outbreak. Reflecting the rootedness to the "Five Shared Values," the explicitly top-down and paternalistic government measures faced little resistance by Singaporeans who were mostly compliant with the quarantine orders because of respect for authority. Consequently, there was little public outcry for restraint on the part of the government for their enactment of "draconian" quarantine laws, as labeled by some foreign media (A. Lee 2003). As Chinese newspaper *Lianhe Zaobao* columnist Lee Huay Leng (2003) suggests in describing the public's consensus with the government:

> Greater liberalization in recent years has seen the emergence of voices critical of
> the government within the country. But during this extraordinary period, there
> has been no querulous voice, no criticism that would shake public morale, in all
> the public feedback on what the government is doing.   (p. 3)

As Lee's comments suggest, the gradual "liberalization" of public discourse, which
was enacted through such programs as *Singapore 21* (1999) and *Remaking Singapore* (2003), laid a solid foundation for the communication strategies to effectively
gain public support for strong social measures during the national health crisis.
This cooperation was in stark contrast to the effervescent public debate over preceding issues such as the transport fare-hikes and importation of foreign-talent.
Accordingly, the implicit trust and faith Singaporeans placed in the government
during times of national crisis were indispensable in the functioning of the social
contract that binds Singaporeans to their leaders and their nation, as a child does
with a parent. Accordingly, the government was credited with solving the health
crisis, thus achieving a resolution (i.e. triumphing over adversity) through mobilizing a nation against the threat of SARS. As *Straits Times'* columnist Janadas
Devan (2003) suggests:

> It is not laissez faire that saves people from burning buildings; it is organised
> courage. It is not the free enterprise system that heals the sick; it is doctors and
> nurses, imbued with public-spiritedness, who get the job done. The free market
> by itself is merely a system of accounting quite ignorant of social values. The glue
> that holds it all together – the civilizational coordinator and guarantor of last
> resort – is government.   (p. 4)

This notion of a social contract also extends to the media-government relationship. As Bokhorst-Heng (2002) suggests, the media are among the social institutions that are closely tied to the government's agenda of nation building. This support was evidenced in the media's spontaneous pro-government stance, providing
the crucial vehicle for the government's communication campaign that helped
bind the nation together as one during the SARS crisis.

    As a result of the actions taken by the government, Singapore's successful stance against SARS and resulting stories of heroism have become a source
of community strength to achieve social cohesion and unity when challenges
emerge in the future. Prime Minister Goh encapsulated the legacy of SARS when
he suggested the "crisis can be turned into something positive" (Ibrahim 2003).
For example, subsequent public communication in Chinese now uses the phrase
weiji for crisis, which combines two characters "wei" (danger) and "ji" (opportunity). In so doing, the discourse on SARS provides the coda or closure to the story
of Singapore's survival, providing additional support for the government's claims
that the crisis had in fact demonstrated how Singapore and Singaporean can come

together and triumph using national strength and character. As Minister Tony Tan suggested:

> As we have fought against SARS, so we must similarly gear ourselves to meet the two other challenges which face Singapore today: terrorism and economic slow-down. . . . If we show the same spirit as we did in the battle against SARS, we will undoubtedly get through this difficult period.   (Ibrahim 2003, p. 6)

Given this analysis of the discourse on SARS, it is possible to see how the government and the media linked situated meanings relating to war to the cultural models of "Five Shared Values" and Confucianism so as to mobilize the nation during the SARS outbreak. For example, the use of war metaphors, and related emotive words such as *battle*, *enemy*, and *heroism*, was already built into contemporary discourse on the "war against terrorism," in which Singapore has been a vocal supporter since September 11, as well as in the discourse about the Bali bombing that occurred just six months before the health crisis emerged. On a broader level, the heroic stories showed individual citizens how they could come together as a community and respond more effectively to such threats by adhering to principles of the "Five Shared Values." Through media reports, the medical community's bravery and sacrifice became tangible signifiers of the core national values emphasizing: nation before community and society above self, family as the basic unit of society, community support and respect for the individual, and consensus not conflict.

In applying Gee's (2002) discourse analysis framework, it is possible to see how the government organized the larger pieces of information that constituted the civic discourse on how Singaporeans should respond as one nation. This organization can be laid out in Gee's (2002) narrative structure of: *setting* (citizen, government and SARS); *catalyst* (life-threatening disease); *crisis* (erosion of core values and a threat to social cohesion), *evaluation* (shared experiences of social responsibility and sacrifice), *resolution* (triumph over adversity), and *coda* (experience builds national strength and character). Together, these components formed a powerful and cohesive communicative framework that helped to mobilize Singaporeans to be socially responsible and make sacrifices for the nation. Consequently, the government now has a more powerful model of what constitutes an ideal Singaporean citizen, one that can be used as another "floating signifier" to galvanize Singaporeans whenever precautions are necessary to secure the nation's future in times of crisis.

Conclusions

The study set out to examine the contribution Singapore's fight against SARS made to the national mythology of "triumph over adversity," given the success of the government's communication program to mobilize the nation's population during the SARS crisis in 2003. Findings indicate that the addition of the themes of "social responsibility" and "sacrifice" within civic discourse strengthened the national mythology because the crisis was not directly linked to the previously defining floating signifier of "economic resilience." In this situation, SARS was constructed through civic discourse as an internal threat, striking directly at the core of Singapore's "Five Shared Values" framework, rather than something external and uncontrollable, such as the 1997 Asian financial crisis or the historically distant riots in the 1960s.

Crucial to this success was the foundation laid by the government through re-working the Confucian ethic into a more appealing and relevant value system. As Tu (1996) argues, Singapore's Confucian movement in the 1980s had realized its aim of sensitizing the country's citizenry to the positive values of their Confucian heritage, albeit in a modified, popularized, and subtly re-worked version found in the "Five Shared Values." Elements of "social responsibility" and "sacrifice" link directly to this hierarchical values framework of nation before community and society above self, family as the basic unit of society, community support and respect for the individual, and consensus not conflict. These values became naturalized and thus tangible for every Singaporean through the stories of real people or "heroes" that the government drew upon to rally public support in the face of adversity caused by SARS. Accordingly, government communication during the health crisis contributed significantly to the enrichment of the self-sustaining mythology of "triumph over adversity," which attempts to tie citizens to national goals. By demonstrating how socially responsible citizens can contribute directly to the nation, the mythology helps Singaporeans to identify with the cultural model of national strength and character exemplified by the heroism of the medical community as a way of reinforcing the ideal values for all Singaporeans. This addition to the mythology of "triumph over adversity" should serve the Singaporean government's future efforts to motivate citizens to be socially responsible to national goals when the next crisis emerges to challenge the city-state's national character.

References

ACNielsen Research. (2003, October 6). Up close and personal: Nielsen Media Research reveals what Singaporeans read, watch and listen. Retrieved November 9, 2003, from http://www.acnielsen.com.sg/news.asp?newsID=134

Barthes, R. (1972). *Mythologies* [trans. by Annette Lavers]. New York: Hill and Wang.

Bokhorst-Heng, W. (2002). Newspapers in Singapore: A mass ceremony in the imagining of the nation. *Media, Culture & Society, 24,* 559–569.

Brown, D. (1993). *Democratization and national identity in East Asia and Southeast Asia.* Singapore: Department of Political Science, National University of Singapore.

Chang, A. (2003, May 31). Singapore is off WHO's SARS list. *Straits Times.* Retrieved September 1, 2003, from Factiva database.

Chua, B. H. (1998). Culture, multiracialism, and national identity in Singapore. In K.-H. Chen (Ed.), *Trajectories: Inter-Asia cultural studies* (pp. 186–205). London: Routledge.

Chua, B. H., & Kuo, E. C. Y. (1995). *The making of a new nation: Communitarian ideology and democracy in Singapore.* London: Routledge.

Chua, M. H. (2004). *A defining moment: How Singapore beat SARS.* Singapore: Ministry of Information, Communication and the Arts.

Devan, J. (2003, April 26). A show of courage, a matter of trust and faith. *Straits Times.* Retrieved September 1, 2003, from Factiva database.

Fairclough, N. (1995). *Media discourse.* London: Edward Arnold.

From bullock carts to budget carriers, via the Concorde. (2004, February 23). *Straits Times.* Retrieved March 10, 2004, from Factiva database.

Gee, J. P. (2002). *An introduction to discourse analysis: Theory and method.* London: Routledge.

Goh, C. T. (2003a, August 17). From the valley to the highlands. National Day Rally Speech by the Prime Minister, Singapore. Retrieved August 30, 2003, from http://app.sprinter.gov.sg/data/pr/2003081707.htm.

Goh, C. T. (2003b, April 22). Fighting SARS together. Open letter by the Prime Minister, Singapore. Retrieved August 30, 2003, from http://app.sprinter.gov.sg/data/pr/2003042204.htm.

Goh, C. T. (2003c, May 1). Prime Minister's May Day message 2003. Retrieved August 30, 2003, from http://app.sprinter.gov.sg/data/pr/2003042908.htm.

Graham, P. (1999). Critical systems theory: A political economy of language, thought, and technology. *Communication Research, 26,* 482–507.

Henson, B. (2003, May 1). WHO praises S'pore's moves to fight virus. *Straits Times.* Retrieved September 1, 2003, from Factiva database.

Ho, K. L. (2000). Prime ministerial leadership and policy-making style in Singapore: Lee Kuan Yew and Goh Chok Tong compared. *Asian Journal of Political Science, 8*(1), 91–123.

Ibrahim, Z. (2003, May 10). PM praises S'poreans for facing up to SARS. *Straits Times.* Retrieved September 1, 2003, from Factiva database.

Khalik, S. (2003, April 7). PM Goh praises 'valiant' doctors and nurses. *Straits Times.* Retrieved September 1, 2003, from Factiva database.

Kluver, R., & Weber, I. (2003). Patriotism and the limits of globalization: Renegotiating citizenship in Singapore. *Journal of Communication Inquiry, 27,* 371–388.

Kuo, E. C. Y. (1996). Confucianism as political discourse in Singapore: The case of an incomplete revitalization movement. In W. Tu. (Ed.), *Confucian traditions in East Asian modernity: Moral education and economic culture in Japan and the Four Mini-Dragons* (pp. 294–309). Cambridge, MA: Harvard University Press.

Lee, A. (2003, April 27). Singapore's SARS moves world's toughest – BBC. *Straits Times*. Retrieved September 1, 2003, from Factiva database.

Lee, H. L. (2003, April 24). SARS – a national response. Ministerial statement in parliament. Retrieved September 1, 2003, from http://www.sars.gov.sg/archive/.

Lee, K. Y. (2000). *From third world to first: The Singapore story, 1965–2000*. Singapore: Times Private Media.

Long, S. (2003, May 11). Singapore at war. *Straits Times*. Retrieved September 1, 2003, from Factiva database.

Mauzy, D. K., & Milne, R. S. (2002). *Singapore politics under the People's Action Party*. London: Routledge.

Media rivals team up to start SARS TV channel. (2003, May 17). *Straits Times*. Retrieved September 1, 2003, from Factiva database.

Remaking Singapore Committee. (2003). *The report of the remaking Singapore Committee: Changing mindsets, deepening relationships*. Singapore: Singapore Government.

Riegel, J. (2002). Confucius. Retrieved September 1, 2003, from http://plato.stanford.edu/archives/fall2002/entries/confucius/

Sim, G. (2003, March 28). Travel dealt blow after blow. *Straits Times*. Retrieved September 1, 2003, from Factiva database.

Singapore 21 Committee. (1999). *Singapore 21: Together, we make the difference*. Singapore: Singapore Government.

Sreenvasan, V. (2004, March 2). SIA's profit recovery set to be good news for staff; Carrier likely to hit $600m target, restore cuts and pay out 15% bonus. *Straits Times*. Retrieved March 10, 2004, from Factiva database.

Straits Times. (2004). About us. Retrieved November 11, 2003, from http://www.straitstimes.com/aboutus/0,1959,00.html

Tu, W. (Ed.). (1996). *Confucian traditions in East Asian modernity: Moral education and economic culture in Japan and the four mini-dragons* (pp. 259–264). Cambridge, MA: Harvard University Press.

World Bank commends Singapore for SARS fight. (2003, May 13). The World Bank East Asia and Pacific Region. Retrieved September 1, 2003 from http://www.sars.gov.sg/archive/World%20Bank.doc

CHAPTER 9

Singapore at war

SARS and its metaphors

Chris Hudson
RMIT University

The spread of SARS in Singapore in early 2003 became a public spectacle in which a deadly illness was metaphorically transmuted into a threat to the integrity of the nation. The "War on SARS" entered the popular imagination in parallel with the war in Iraq. The military war on terrorism circulated in the same discursive space as the biological war on disease, thereby invoking the language of military strength, a community united in adversity, the defence of national borders, and the threat of a pestilence that had the potential to kill the economy. Singapore became an ideological battleground where disease was central to an imagery of the fear of social disorder created by an unknown enemy. This chapter examines the ways in which SARS acquired metaphorically charged meaning beyond the basic epidemiological concerns. A reformulation of Singapore's national identity as a fragile and vulnerable nation served to generate mass ideological mobilization, made possible through discursive spectacles in the national media. Successful eradication of the disease became a "defining moment" in the history of Singapore, and brought about a resurgence of national identity.

Introduction

Not long after the first SARS patients were admitted to Singapore's Tan Tock Seng hospital in the first quarter of 2003, a new aesthetics of nation appeared in Singapore's public discourse, one that transformed SARS from a pathogen of the human body into an enemy of the body politic. This chapter examines the ways in which the threat of a physical disease was reinterpreted metaphorically to become the enemy of a just society – one which would infect not only a number of individuals, but would also pathologize the nation itself. During the SARS crisis, Singapore society was both medicalized and militarized. This not only enabled the mass mobilization of Singaporean bodies to fight the physical disease, but also the mass ideological mobilization of Singaporean minds. The large-scale organization required to isolate and contain the physical disease, and the strategic textual practices that were employed to accomplish that task, united the vulnerable bodies of Singaporeans in an orderly system of commitment to the survival of a putatively vulnerable nation. These strategies appeared as an extended spectacle of nation, apparently as powerful in its potential to unite as other traditional spectacles of nation such as the National Day Parade.

By the time SARS had been brought under control in Singapore, 238 people had been infected and 33 people had died as a consequence. That SARS was a highly dangerous illness is not in dispute; nor is the speed and efficiency with which clinical and prophylactic measures were used to prevent the spread of the disease. This chapter will, however, explore the ways in which SARS in Singapore acquired meaning beyond epidemiological concerns to create a parallel reality of a nation at war. In Singapore in 2003, disease was as much a political event as a medical event, and the boundary markers of the nation and of national duty were the subject of the discourse.

A useful starting point for understanding the ideological and political environment of Singapore, in which anxiety about vulnerability has become a dominant mode of imagining the nation, is to consider the power of metaphor both to reveal and conceal meaning. I will discuss certain aspects of Singapore society as a prelude to an analysis of the SARS crisis. I will then highlight three salient features of the social construction of SARS in Singapore, that is: the politicization of personal health behaviour as part of the militarization of the nation in its fight against SARS; the obscuring of potentially dangerous cultural and political diversity within a framework in which the state represents its interests as consistent with the interests of individual citizens; and the reinvigoration of nationalism, coupled with the reinscription of Singapore's future as a physically and economically healthy, internationally respected and globally connected nation.

The chapter is divided into the following broad areas: methodological considerations, the media and metaphor, the ideological environment, the discursive field created by the SARS crisis, and a conclusion which considers the importance of spectacle for the promotion of national unity.

Methodological considerations

My approach in this chapter is to examine the narrative address of the nation, as Bhabha (1990) suggests we should if we are to understand the ideological apparatus of state power. The series of discursive events which emerged during the SARS crisis can be thought of as a chapter in the ongoing "text of nation" – an episode which deployed figurative language as much as scientific facts for its construction of the meaning of illness. Chew and Kramer-Dahl (1999) recommend textual analysis in order to understand discursive strategies in Singapore which reinforce national culture while articulating responses to political or physical events. They argue for the "disentangling of multiple layers of context, of subtle traces of subtext as well as historical and synchronic intertexts of texts of Singapore culture" (Chew & Kramer-Dahl 1999, p. 3).

Since Chua (1995) has argued that Singapore's national identity is the result of its discursive practices, an appropriate method, it seems, is one which discloses these discursive practices. Accordingly, I will examine the ways in which textual representations of the SARS crisis, as they emerged in a variety of public discourses, were instrumental in framing a renewed sense of nationhood and urgency in the face of a common enemy. The complicity between the press and politics is central to understanding the ways in which illness was represented as an enemy of the nation. My primary focus, therefore, is on the mass media and the public statements of community leaders and politicians.

It is now axiomatic to say that cultural and national identities are invented and constructed through discursive means. Anderson (1991) has encouraged us to think of the nation as an imagined political community. The nation has to be imagined as a community because we cannot be acquainted with everybody in it; and it is imagined as both limited and sovereign (Anderson 1991, pp. 6–7). Anderson explored the origins of national consciousness and concluded that print capitalism laid the basis for it. The press is a preeminent site for the production of the narrative address of nation, and it can be both populist and instrumental, as Anderson has argued.

For Anderson (1991) the nation is a set of cultural representations that provides the means for citizens to imagine the ways in which they belong to the collective. Concerted attempts to invent a national identity and construct a mode of thinking through which the collective could be imagined have been well recognized in Singapore (for example, Ban, Pakir, & Tong 2004; Chew & Kramer-Dahl 1999) – a state whose formative characteristics include a relatively short history as a collective with an identity, and a manageably-sized multiethnic population living in a limited and insular geographical space.

While the mass media can provide the site for the production of national identity and impart a unity of purpose amongst readers, we can gain a more nuanced and sophisticated understanding of the processes if we also consider the informing premise of Bhabha's (1994) work on the nation. For him, the overriding feature of the nation is that it is an irredeemably plural modern space, in which national unity consists in the continual displacement of the anxiety engendered by this plurality (p. 149). Representations of national unity can be seen as attempts to overcome the anxiety of confronting uncontrolled difference. The SARS crisis in Singapore presented the opportunity to displace some anxieties associated with a plural and culturally diverse society. It was made possible through powerful discourses which appealed to citizens' understanding of national unity, as much as to a shared fear of the illness.

The media and metaphor

The media in Singapore had a dual role in the process of the social construction of SARS. They were at once transparent and honest in reporting empirical facts about the nature and spread of the disease; but they were also complicit in the deployment of strategic ambiguities for political ends. The "War on SARS" became a mode of representation that paradoxically limited possible understanding while, at the same time, expanded its social meaning to encompass a political narrative of nationhood. Susan Sontag's (1978, 1989) essays on the use of figurative devices in descriptions of illness draw attention to the way in which metaphor can be used to create meanings that can be detached from scientific realities and reconfigured for political and ideological purposes (Baehr 2006). Other writers have also examined the way in which societies have imagined disease and the narrative possibilities of epidemics (Gilman 1988; Larson, Nerlich, & Wallis 2005; Rosenberg 1995; Vrettos 1995).

Lakoff and Johnson (1980) argue that the systematicity that allows us to comprehend one aspect of a concept in terms of another – the essence of metaphor – also provides for concealment of meaning. Metaphor, they argue, can "highlight or hide" (p. 10). The metaphor of war was systematically deployed during the SARS crisis in Singapore to the extent that it became the structuring principle that dominated all public discussions about it. In Lakoff and Johnson's terms, the concept of illness was metaphorically structured in terms of war (p. 14).

In the absence of a real war in the short history of post-colonial Singapore, the war on SARS became the defining moment of military glory – creating a parallel reality encompassing a moral universe of national duty and heroism. SARS went beyond its nature as an illness to inspire a spectacle of national pride to unite all Singaporeans. It highlighted the concerted and unified effort people took to control the spread of disease, while at the same time it hid from view Bhabha's irredeemably plural space of nationhood.

The political and ideological environment

Singapore has been ruled by the People's Action Party since 1959 when the former British colony was granted internal self-government. Since independence in 1965, it has had only three Prime Ministers. Lee Kuan Yew led the country until 1990, when he was succeeded by Goh Chok Tong. Lee's son Lee Hsien Loong was instated as the Prime Minister on 12 August 2004.

Policies of social control have always been an important feature of Singapore's economic development. One pre-eminent means of social control has been to create a climate of fear. Histories of modern Singapore are often narratives of a fraught beginning followed by decades of anxiety and fear. Singapore is imagined as having embarked on a difficult journey (Ban 1992) as a vulnerable and reluctant small nation after the traumatic expulsion from the union with Malaysia in 1965 (Lee 1998, p. 2). The standard narrative of nation is a series of struggles against hostile forces and untoward circumstances (Drysdale 1996).

Clammer (1998) echoes other observers such as Lingle (1996) when he calls Singapore a "society of fear" in which internal factors are as much a source of anxiety as the external Other. The rhetoric of threat to a vulnerable nation, with its people constituting its only resource, is a frequently conjured trope of nationhood in Singapore.

If imaginings of the nation are dominated by the idea of fragility and vulnerability, fear itself becomes a resource to be used in nation-building and social control. In the decades since independence, anxieties have emerged in discourses concerning the fear of communism, of a slow economy, of too high a population increase, of racial violence, of an environment dominated by hostile Muslims, of Westernisation, of liberal values, of too low a population, of foreign workers, of drug abuse, of lack of commitment to competitiveness, of creeping welfarism, of financial meltdown. Anxieties have also centred on the body, so that crises arise out of the threat of exogamy, miscegenation, graduate women remaining unmarried, and most recently of the global spread of disease. The repeatability of such varied but consistent menaces affords narrative authority and makes available for the national imagination an almost infinitely expandable discursive space of fear of the threatening external Other. In Singapore, a society comprised of a racial mélange of Chinese, Indians and Malays, this overlaps with an internal enemy: the Other of a Chinese patriarchal polity. The boundaries of the nation and the internal divisions between groups categorised as Other – Bhabha's irredeemable plurality – are maintained by recourse to discourses of uncertainty and crisis.

Birch (1993) has described a myth of nationhood in Singapore whose central metaphorical construct is the vulnerability of the nation. Its predominant imagery is the crisis, which achieves its material existence through "staging" in the state-controlled media. According to Birch (1993):

> Certainly within Singapore the very maintenance of the discourse of crisis is one of the main strategies adopted by the Singapore government to maintain its ideology of control, anchor its people to the nation and create a climate of domestic uncertainty about the fragility of the state and the economy.   (p. 75)

In Singapore, the local discourse of fear linked to the global discourse of epidemic, reconfigured the culture of anxiety, enhanced it by enlarging its frame to the regional and global, and brought about a resurgence of nationalism. What was important in the discursive uses of SARS in Singapore was the location of disease; it was not just an atypical pneumonia caused by a coronavirus that randomly found bodies to host it, but it invaded the space of the nation, and travelled internationally.

Singapore was already a militarized society before the SARS crisis. Militarism is an integral part of the national culture, as the display of military hardware at any National Day Parade will confirm. Conscription for National Service (NS) was introduced in 1967, and all young men serve two or more years in the armed forces. NS is compulsory only for men, and it has become a site for the struggle over citizenship and legitimacy as a national subject. Heng and Devan (1995) identify two types of nationalism in Singapore:

> A sexualized, separate species of nationalism, in other words, was being advocated for women: as patriotic duty for men grew out of the barrel of a gun (phallic nationalism, the wielding of a surrogate technology of the body in national defense), so it would grow, for women, out of the recesses of the womb (uterine nationalism, the body as a technology of defense wielded by the nation). Men bearing arms and women bearing children.   (p. 201)

One frame through which these deeply gendered interpretations of national duty could be articulated and united as an ensemble of available ways of becoming a participating citizen, was the concept of Total Defence. The government website promoting the concept says:

> Many people think of Total Defence as a defence strategy or plan that is rolled out only during times of war. But it is more than that. Total Defence is about the different things that we can do everyday in every sector of our society to strengthen our resilience as a nation. When we take National Service seriously, participate in civil emergency exercises, upgrade ourselves and learn new skills, build strong bonds with different races and religions, and feel the pride of being Singaporean, we contribute to Total Defence.   (Singapore Government 2004a)

The policy of Total Defence which first emerged in the public sphere in 1984, incorporates not only Military Defence, but Economic, Psychological, Social and Civil Defence. According to the government website, "the five elements work together as a comprehensive defence strategy for Singapore." Total Defence has interpellated every Singaporean into a militarized milieu with slogans such as "*Without You*, our doors might be left wide open"; "*Without You*, a threat might go unnoticed" (Singapore Government 2004b); "Total Defence: There's a part for everyone" (Singapore Government 2004c). With the emergence of this discourse, a whole society could be militarized, and a climate of defensiveness and alert to potential threat maintained, even in times of prosperity and peace.

There are also other aspects of Singapore society on which state controlled discourses can draw for their potency, including particular kinds of social relationships. Eminent Singapore sociologist, Chua Beng Huat (1995) has termed Singapore a "communitarian democracy" (p. 185), that is, a non-liberal democracy where collective well-being is safeguarded by good government by honourable leaders. In this system there is a conflation of state and society, made possible through the notion that their interests coincide. Rather than a democracy based on the liberalism and personal freedom of the Western model, "the conflation of state/society justifies interventions in all spheres of social life, rationalized as pre-emptive interventions which 'ensure' the collective well-being, as measures of good government rather than abuses of civil rights" (Chua 1995, p. 187). Because every level of daily life is drawn into this encompassing realm, almost every daily action is available for politicization, including the contracting of disease. A polity of this nature, where intervention into the social is seen as its primary method, requires its authority, as Mules (1999) has pointed out, to be asserted *directly* (p. 74) into the national public sphere. The media is the prime site for this intervention.

When the citizen is directly addressed in this manner, he or she is called into being as a subject of the state who will participate in the system for reproducing the conditions of production and power relations. It is a ritualized form of address to citizens, according to Althusser (1971), which represents the subject's material relationship to the state. In an ideological environment in which the citizens are familiar with the state's expectations of them and where their material relationship to the state is seemingly unambiguous ("Without you!"), the master text of the battle against SARS could reiterate and reinforce the necessity of this relationship, constitute people as subjects, and define their subject position.

It was into this ideological milieu that the first SARS case found its way in early 2003. All these strands in the narrative address of the nation came together during the ensuing crisis. The renewed militarization of society with a concomitant politicization of individual actions, the promotion of putative national unity in the face of intransigent plurality, the conflation of the interests of the state with the interests of the citizen, and the emergence of Singapore as a player on the world stage in the fight against global epidemic, all appeared as elements in the social construction of SARS.

The discursive field of SARS

This section will examine the discursive terrain in which these elements were arranged. Firstly, from the outset when the initial SARS cases appeared, a repertoire of military metaphors animated the discourses. For example, on April 24, then Deputy Prime Minister Lee Hsien Loong declared the country "officially at war, with battles being waged on three fronts – public health, the economy and society" (*Straits Times*, May 11, 2003). Similarly, the Home Affairs Minister Wong Kan Seng was dubbed the Donald Rumsfeld of the SARS wars (*Straits Times*, May 11) when he was charged with leading a nine-member inter-ministry Task Force. Senior Minister of State (Transport, Information and the Arts), Khaw Boon Wan, who became known as the SARS Czar was put in charge of a Combat Team of junior ministers. Moreover, personal conduct associated with illness was also politicized. Minister of State (Education and Manpower), Ng Eng Heng, said that:

> Infected people are carriers of "bombs" attached on them by the Sars "enemy" and these explosives can go off if they do not seek help . . . The Sars combat unit is prepared to fight the enemy, but Singaporeans, please don't shoot and kill your own troops. Be truthful, be responsible.　　(*Straits Times,* February, 2, 2004)

Straits Times correspondent, Zubaidah Ibrahim, noted that Singaporeans "have had to wrestle with a series of difficulties – from the terror threat exposed by September 11, attacks in 2001, the Bali bomb blasts last year, which sent shivers down spines in the region, and now SARS" (*Straits Times*, May 10, 2003). She reported that at the end of a visit to the US, PM Goh Chok Tong told a gathering that:

> Every single Singaporean is a soldier in the fight against Sars. We have armed every household with a thermometer. That's a weapon. We involved them in this fight against a common enemy. If we succeed in controlling the problem, out of all this, we are going to see a stronger Singapore because we are all in this fight together.　　(*Straits Times*, May 10, 2003)

Dr. Ong Jin Ee, writing in the *Straits Times*, linked the disease with a real war:

> With a military war raging in Iraq and a biological war raging in Singapore against severe acute respiratory syndrome (SARS) we are in need of something that will encourage our hearts.　　(*Straits Times*, March 28, 2003)

The government made an announcement that the whole country would be put on alert on March 15, 2003, and then began to mobilize the nation. Measures taken to control the disease were carried out not just with military precision, but by the military itself. National servicemen were put on duty at Changi Airport to screen visitors arriving from SARS affected areas, in the hope that they could "bludgeon the enemy into submission." The military was mobilized to distribute thermometers to 1.1 million homes. The Infectious Diseases Act was amended to give the military the power to use any means necessary to stop the spread, including jailing and fining quarantine breakers. It used two main strategies to monitor and control the population: contact tracing (searching for those who had had contact with infected people), and the taking of temperatures. Temperature checks were carried out at all land, air and sea entry points into Singapore. The taking of temperatures became a ritual as stallholders and their assistants at 134 wet markets were required to take their temperatures twice a day. An arsenal of thermal scanners, electronic cameras, electronic tagging, and naming and shaming of people who broke quarantine orders was introduced.

A SARS Task Force was set up in every community to spread the message of public hygiene, under the management of Wong Kan Seng, the Minister for Home Affairs, and deputy chairman of the People's Association. The PA, the statutory board that is in charge of 2,000 grassroots organizations, played a key role in containing the outbreak. It was mobilized at short notice to help with the "contact chasing" of 2,400 workers at the Pasir Panjang wholesale market from where the disease had apparently spread. Emergency housing was made available to those who were diagnosed as infected. Surgical masks, gloves and gowns were distributed on a mass scale to hospital workers. People visiting hospitals were issued with card sized censors to track their movements. Cisco guards[1] were employed on contact tracing and serving home quarantine orders. In late March 2003, schools and colleges were shut down for two weeks and Pasir Panjang wholesale market was closed. SARS invaded the field of popular culture, with local sitcom character Phua Chu Kang singing songs about hygiene and socially responsible behaviour, and radio and television talk shows devoting air time to it.

Secondly, the discourse of war provided space to refocus attention on the good and honourable leader who would place himself at the disposal of the community to ensure the welfare of all. Drawing on the modes of communication and the strategy of direct address, described by Mules (1999), and the ideology of the communitarian democracy, political leaders, inscribed themselves as ordinary citizens and became an integral component of the ideological war. This strategic move was

---

1.   Cisco is a private security company which was established as a statutory board of the Ministry of Home Affairs.

able to reinforce the idea that every citizen at every level was part of a national team fighting a common enemy, regardless of social status, income or class.

The parliamentary debate on SARS was televised live. Lee Kuan Yew shared his family's close encounter with the disease; security guards took temperatures of MPs at parliament house; Wong Kan Seng, head of the SARS War team and Minister for Home Affairs, made public his personal management of the self in the fight against SARS:

> The only thing that has changed is that my family and I take our temperatures every day, religiously. I take my temperature after I wake up and brush my teeth.
> (*Straits Times*, May 18, 2003)

On May 3, 2003, PM Goh, along with ten cabinet and junior ministers, addressed 1,800 grassroots and community leaders at Kallang Theatre. He recalled the communitarian society when he spoke directly to citizens, reducing the symbolic distance between himself and the community, and, in a masculine paradigm of citizenship, exhorted all Singaporeans to involve themselves in the surveillance of others:

> In the early days we did not understand how Sars was spread, so individuals went out, and spread Sars without knowing that they were doing so. But from now on, there is no excuse for anyone in Singapore not to know the part he has to play and that when he has a fever, he may be a potential infector. So the message is a simple one. All of us as ordinary citizens, you and I, have a part to fight Sars and keep Singapore cool. . . . Beyond acting responsibly, people must take steps to stop an irresponsible person from spreading Sars.   (*Straits Times*, May 3, 2003)

In a move which further reduced the distance between state and citizen, Goh Chok Tong spoke directly to the people of Singapore in an open letter on April 23, 2003. Deputy Director of the Institute of Policy Studies, Arun Mahizhnan, praised Goh's letter, calling it a "key moment" and "quintessentially Goh" for the way in which it reached out in a direct and personal way to every Singaporean (*Straits Times*, May 10, 2003). The *Straits Times* reported that this had earned him the epithet "the Rudy Giuliani of Sars" (May 11, 2003).

At its peak, there were almost daily press conferences during which commanders announced the latest casualty figures, paralleling the American television briefings on the war in Iraq. Politicians and community leaders were televised publicly having their temperatures taken. Tan Tock Seng Hospital had all other services suspended and it was decreed SARS central (*Straits Times*, May 11, 2003). Colonel Goh Chye Kim an IDSS[2] military analyst said that fierce frontline

---

2. Institute of Defence and Strategic Studies.

fighting was backed up by an intense media campaign akin to wartime information operations aimed at winning the hearts and minds of people and getting them to do the right thing. The *Straits Times* called SARS Singapore's September 11 (May 11, 2003). One article encapsulated the mobilization of Singapore, and extended the metaphors of illness to the economy:

> Singapore has been metamorphosed into Thermometer Nation. The economy is wheezing away, more than 3,000 residents have been quarantined and the death toll lurks at 27. The new national must-have accessory is a fever-free sticker.
>
> What started out as Health Minister Lim Hng Kiang's one-man battle has revved into an all-out war, one that has engaged virtually every minister and even statutory boards like the People's Association.
>
> From the national servicemen roped in to screen visitors from Sars-affected areas at Changi Airport to the security guard at Parliament House taking temperatures of MPs to the grassroots leaders pressed into service as a contact tracer, the war effort involving thousands of Singaporeans in a 24-hour, seven days a week campaign that has multiple enemies: the virus, fear, ignorance, social irresponsibility, an ailing economy and international perceptions.
>
> For more than a month now, the government has been knee deep in the trenches, mounting Singapore's biggest shock and awe offensive in peace time. The battle-lines to isolate, contain and kill the bug – with whatever means necessary – have been drawn.   (*Straits Times*, May 11, 2003)

Taking your own temperature regularly, staying healthy, and remaining SARS-free became a national duty. A new nationalism was born which united gender, race and class: out of the crisis grew a sort of "corporate wellness" nationalism, conflating a healthy body with a healthy body politic. The welfare of every person became synonymous with the welfare of the nation. The new national rhetoric was able to conceal the contested gender divide – encapsulated by Heng and Devan's (1995) description of the phallic nationalism/uterine nationalism dichotomy – while highlighting the unity of purpose of the nation.

The unity imagined through the struggle against a common enemy was able to displace anxiety about pluralism and cultural diversity, onto anxiety about the illness. SARS had the ability to unite ethnic communities previously divided on political and religious issues, and to erase difference in the cause of nationhood. The *Straits Times* reported that Lee Hsien Loong had observed that although Muslim Singaporeans viewed the Iraq war differently, this did not mean they were less committed than anyone else to the fight against SARS:

> Malay-Muslim doctors, nurses and other health care workers have stood bravely in the front lines of the battle against the virus. And Malay-Muslim policemen, soldiers and personnel in the Singapore Civil Defence Force have carried out

> their duties in guarding the entry points and key installations, as part of the na-
> tion's multi-racial security force. *(Straits Times*, May 25, 2003)

Religious differences were erased, to be obscured by the image of a nation united against a common enemy.

Thirdly, Singapore was able to imagine itself as a nation strengthened and revitalized by the SARS crisis. It helped invent a bright future for the nation by reinvigorating support for the government and by providing a field of comparisons, both to reconfigure illness as an enemy equal to a hostile state and to elevate Singapore's place in regional geopolitics. Dr. Andrew Tan an analyst from IDSS, notes:

> What impressed me most was the Government's vigour and thoroughness in tracking down the chain of transmission in order to contain it. Not many countries can do this successfully. China would have huge problems because of its size. Hong Kong could, but instead failed to do as well due to this lack of political will and decisive leadership. Such a response ... shows that in a real war, the Government will strike back hard if attacked, whether it is by an invisible virus or an unfriendly belligerent state. *(Straits Times*, May 11, 2003)

The SARS crisis could offer an opportunity to renew citizens' relationship to the state, and promote the idea of social equality. Dr. Tan Chi Chiu, Singapore International Foundation's director, said:

> International acclaim has been well deserved and will not go unnoticed by people. They can compare the quality of governments in different countries in a very direct way, through government responses, since Sars is a great leveler ... Confidence in the Government and approval ratings must be at an all time high right now. If the PAP government needed to accumulate credits with the people by the next election, and the cupboard seemed a bit bare lately, the Sars crisis made it possible for it to make good in a major way. ... We have seldom felt more united as a people, with the blurring of the Us and Them syndrome with respect to relating to the government. *(Straits Times*, May 11, 2003)

A government previously condemned for its secrecy, was praised for its transparency. For people who worried that the SARS crisis might vindicate the government's autocratic management of the country, SARS could offer a social transformation and a new beginning:

> When the fighting on the front stops, the reconstruction of a new post-Sars social order must begin. Most hope that the collective way the Sars War is being fought will provide an impetus for a new, more equal and respectful partnership in government. *(Straits Times*, May 11, 2003)

The crisis also had longer term effects on the revitalization of national sentiment. The "Singapore's OK" campaign, a vehicle for the 80 SARS Task Forces, celebrated its first year of existence by renewing its commitment to the nation. Minister Lim Swee Say said:

> Basically we look at "Singapore's OK" not as 100-m dash, not that it started with Sars and now that Sars is over, it will end with Sars. Instead, we'll look at "Singapore's OK" as a marathon, a never-ending race, an unending battle against unknown viruses, unknown diseases.   (See 2004)

Some of the these SARS Task Forces have extended their possible life span and usefulness to the community by restructuring themselves as Emergency Preparedness Groups or Environmental Hygiene and Public Health Safety Committees.

A war produces heroes, and becomes an epochal event in the narrative of any nation. The war on SARS in Singapore created a moral universe, in which health care workers became known as "SARS warriors" and were publicly acknowledged for their dedication and valour (*Straits Times*, July 4, 2003). Letters taking up the bigger questions of the universal need for heroic figures appeared in the press:

> we feel proud of doctors, nurses and health-care workers there [at Tan Tock Seng Hospital] . . . The world is short of heroes and heroines and their contributions should not go unnoticed.
>
> (Dr. Ong Jin Ee, letter to the *Straits Times*, March 28, 2003)

In his National Day Message, 2003, Prime Minister Goh also pointed to the everyday heroism of citizens and the potential of fear to unite the nation. Fear became a historical, even epochal, event. He linked the danger of the epidemic to more general threats to the nation such as the faltering economy, the competition from cheap labour elsewhere, and regional terrorism:

> I am proud of us Singaporeans, for our unity and our conduct in fighting SARS. SARS is a deadly disease. But we fought it bravely and smartly. The threat was common to all of us, and every Singaporean took up arms and closed ranks. We stood shoulder to shoulder, regardless of colour or creed. We lived up to our National Pledge . . . Now, we need that same solidarity and spirit to deal with another challenge – getting our economy healthy and strong again . . . We have suffered successive blows in the last six years. First, the Asian financial crisis. Then, the recession in 2001 and the Jemaah Islamiyah terror plot. And this year, SARS . . .
>
> But take heart. We have faced many storms before, and we have always pulled through. This time, our recovery has taken longer than usual because of a series of unfortunate events. But I am confident that we can overcome our problems, and grow again . . .

> Our performance against SARS has reinforced investors' confidence in us. They noted our swift and total response, and the partnership between the Government and the people. Companies and businessmen are impressed with our ability to overcome shocks to our system. They have told us that they intend to do more in Singapore.
>
> But they have also cautioned us to trim our costs.
>
> The reason is simple: we are up against strong competition from lower-cost countries . . . We also face the same challenge as developed economies like the US, which are seeing the migration of white-collar jobs to India, the Philippines and Thailand.
>
> My fellow Singaporeans, our future is in our hands.
>
> Today, Singapore is a vibrant economy, and a safe and comfortable home for all seasons. The country has thrived because we made difficult but right decisions, and implemented them with resolve. Singapore may not be perfect, but it is our own flesh and blood. This is our country. This is our home. Here, we decide our own destiny. We must never give up on making Singapore even better.
>
> (Singapore Government 2003a)

Goh was also able to unite the global with the local, and the everyday with the epochal, by announcing Singapore's relocation onto the international stage. The nation itself was inscribed as hero:

> When I visited President George Bush in May, he complimented Singapore for having dealt with SARS in a constructive, disciplined and transparent way. The World Health Organisation, too, was impressed. It has formally invited Singapore to be a full member of its global alert and response network. As a full member, Singapore would join a group of select countries which provides experts to help the WHO when infectious diseases break out around the world. So what was it that impressed the international community? First, it was our large reservoir of courage.   (Singapore Government 2003b)

On July 22, 2004, Goh launched a new book on SARS entiltled *A Defining Moment – How Singapore Beat Sars* written by *Straits Times* correspondent Chua Mui Hoong. He said:

> A "defining moment" is more than the title of a new book on Sars. It also captures the essence of what Singapore went through and how the country and people emerged stronger from it . . . the story of the Sars outbreak, our suffering and our fears, and how Singapore contained and beat Sars is a defining moment in our nation's history.   (*Straits Times*, July 25, 2004)

He continued the narrative of the way in which SARS defined the nation in his National Day Rally Speech. Recalling Singapore's history of struggle, he said:

Take a step back into the 60s. Singaporeans felt a similar sense of hopelessness and foreboding then . . . Today, Singapore again faces physical and economic threats. We have to deal with terrorism and SARS . . . unemployment is rising . . . Can we turn Singapore around like Prime Minister Lee did in the 60s? My answer is, yes . . . we have the resources to pull through our problems. More importantly, we have the will. If you have any doubts, look at our performance against SARS . . .

A crisis reveals the true character of a people. Singaporeans passed the SARS test with distinction. We were at war with SARS. To overcome the enemy, we knew we had to work together as a nation. And we did. We closed ranks and stood with each other. We helped each other without regard for race, religion or social position. During this crisis, I saw a national spirit I have never seen before. Our country bonded with stout hearts, tenacity and determination. SARS did not break Singapore, it made us stronger . . .   (Singapore Government 2003c)

Conclusion

The spread of SARS in Singapore became a public spectacle, in which illness was inscribed as a threat to the integrity of the nation. The military war on terrorism and the biological war on disease circulated in the same discursive space, imbricating narratives of military strength, a community united in adversity, the defence of national borders, and the threat of a pestilence that had the potential to kill the economy. It was able to mobilize the nation and renew the relationship between state and subject in a communitarian democracy. Finally, it was able to provide the discursive means by which Singapore could imagine itself in a bright future as a nation of global significance, with an economy and society even more vigorous and successful than before. Despite the deaths it caused, SARS became a positive, nation-building experience for Singapore.

If we recall Birch's (1993) understanding of Singapore as a society which "stages" crises in the media, we can see that SARS, while in reality a dangerous disease, was also a "staged event." It was so intensively focussed on by the mass media that it went beyond its medical significance to achieve "an excess of meaning." The war metaphor, which was universally used to describe the context of the illness, restricted alternative understandings for most people. At the same time, however, it provided an extravagance of meaning through the logic of its continued repetition. It introduced fear, heroes, victory, public spiritedness, transparent government processes, honest media, and a united community into the ontological field; but it also obscured the increased surveillance, militarization, authoritarianism, race and gender difference, and disunity. As a "staged" crisis it was a crucial feature of the ongoing spectacle of regenerated nationalism.

As Debord (1995) has argued, the political economy of modern societies represents itself in an immense accumulation of spectacles. Indeed, the spectacle is so integral and powerful a feature of the modern conditions of production, and of the reproduction of ideology, that the spectacle appears as society itself and the key locus of an imagined unity:

> The spectacle appears at once as society itself, as a part of society and as a means of unification. As a part of society, it is that sector where all attention, all consciousness, converges. (p. 12)

The spectacle of the war on SARS culminated in a defining moment for the nation. The moment, however, went beyond the significance of the control of the disease and victory in the war; the moment achieved its greatest potency when the anxiety engendered by plurality was temporarily displaced by the spectacle of unity. Perhaps the greatest defining moments in any nation are those in which national unity is highlighted and potentially disunifying forces are hidden.

References

Althusser, L. (1971). Ideology and ideological state apparatuses. In *Lenin and philosophy and other essays* (pp. 127–186). New York and London: Monthly Review Press.

Anderson, B. (1983). *Imagined communities. Reflections on the origin and spread of nationalism.* London: Verso.

Baehr, P. (2006). Susan Sontag, battle language and the Hong Kong SARS outbreak of 2003. *Economy and Society, 35,* 42–64.

Ban, K. C. (1992). Narrating imagination. In K. C. Ban, A. Pakir, & C. K. Tong (Eds.), *Imagining Singapore* (pp. 1–15). Singapore: Times Academic Press.

Ban, K. C., Pakir, A., & Tong, C. K. (Eds.). (1992). *Imagining Singapore.* Singapore: Times Academic Press.

Bhabha, H. K. (1994). *The location of culture.* London: Routledge.

Birch, D. (1993). Staging crises: Media and citizenship. In G. Rodan (Ed.), *Singapore changes guard: Social, political and economic directions in the 1990s* (pp. 72–83). New York: Longman Cheshire.

Chew, P. G.-L., & Kramer-Dahl, A. (Eds.). (1999). *Reading culture. Textual practices in Singapore.* Singapore: Times Academic Press.

Chua, B. H. (1995). *Communitarian ideology and democracy in Singapore.* London: Routledge.

Clammer, J. (1998). *Race and state in independent Singapore.* Aldershot: Ashgate.

Debord, G. (1995). *The society of the spectacle.* New York: Zone Books.

Drysdale, J. (1996). *Singapore: Struggle for success.* Singapore: Times Books International.

Gilman, S. L. (1988). *Disease and representation: Images of illness from madness to AIDS.* Ithaca and London: Cornell University Press.

Heng, G., & Devan, J. (1995). State fatherhood: The politics of nationalism, sexuality and race in Singapore. In A. Ong & M. Peletz (Eds.), *Bewitching women, pious men: Gender and body politics in Southeast Asia* (pp. 195–216). Berkeley: University of California Press.

Hill, M., & Fee, L. K. (Eds.). (1995). *The politics of nation building and citizenship in Singapore.* London: Routledge.

Juan, C. S. (1995). *Singapore: My home too.* Singapore: Chee Soon Juan.

Lakoff, G., & Johnson, M. (1980). *Metaphors we live by.* Chicago and London: University of Chicago Press.

Larson, B. M. H., Nerlich, G., & Wallis, P. (2005). Metaphors and biorisks: The war on infectious diseases and invasive species. *Science Communication, 26*, 243–268.

Lee, H. L. (1998). Singapore of the future. In A. Mahizhnan & T. Y. Lee (Eds.), *Singapore: Re-engineering success* (pp. 2–9). Singapore: Oxford University Press.

Leung, P. C., & Ooi, E. E. (2003). *SARS war: Combating the disease.* Singapore: World Scientific.

Lingle, C. (1996). *Singapore's authoritarian capitalism: Asian values, free market illusions, and political dependency.* Barcelona: Edicions Sirocco, S.L.

Mahizhnan, A., & Lee, T. Y. (Eds.). (1998). *Singapore: Re-engineering success.* Singapore: Oxford University Press.

Mules, W. (1999). Globalising discourses: The Flor Contemplacion affair. In P. G. L. Chew & A. Kramer-Dahl (Eds.), *Reading culture. Textual practices in Singapore* (pp. 71–82). Singapore: Times Academic Press.

Rodan, G. (Ed.). (1993). *Singapore changes guard: Social, political and economic directions in the 1990s.* New York: Longman Cheshire.

Rosenberg, C. F. (1992). *Explaining epidemics and other studies in the history of medicine.* Cambridge: Cambridge University Press.

See, B. (2004). *Singapore's OK campaign here to stay, as it celebrates first year.* Retrieved June 12, 2004, from http://www.channelnewsasia.com/stories/singaporelocalnews/view/89700/1/.html.

Singapore Government. (2003a). *National day message.* Retrieved January 27, 2005, from http://www.channelnewsasia.com/nd2003/message/msg_eng.htm.

Singapore Government. (2003b). *Prime minister's national day rally speech.* Retrieved January 27, 2005, from http://www.channelnewsasia.com/nd2003/rally/rally/_eng1.htm.

Singapore Government. (2003c). *From the valley to the highlands – speech by Prime Minister Goh Chok Tong at the national day rally on 17 August 2003.* Retrieved January 27, 2004, from http://www.gov.sg/nd?ND03.htm.

Singapore Government. (2004a). *Total defence.* Retrieved September 3, 2004, from http://www.totaldefence.org/sg/totaldefence/overview.html.

Singapore Government. (2004b). *Total defence.* Retrieved September 3, 2004, from http://www.totaldefence.org/sg/totaldefence/tdlogo.html.

Singapore Government. (2004c). *Total defence.* Retrieved September 3, 2004, from http://totaldefence.org.sg/adgallery/adgallery_print_2004.html.

Sontag, S. (1978). *Illness as metaphor.* New York: Farrar, Straus and Giroux.

Sontag, S. (1989). *AIDS and its metaphors.* New York: Farrar, Straus and Giroux.

Vrettos, A. (1995). *Somatic fictions: Imagining illness in Victorian culture.* Stanford, CA: Stanford University Press.

CHAPTER 10

Reporting an emerging epidemic in Taiwan

Journalists' experiences of SARS coverage*

Mei-Ling Hsu
National Chengchi University

The performance of the mainstream news media during the SARS epidemic, particularly their treatment of risk-related information, raised heated criticism from the government, academia, and public in Taiwan. This study examines journalists' perceptions and experiences in covering the SARS epidemic. Based on in-depth interviews with eight medical journalists from the mainstream news media in June and July 2003, the study addresses the following issues: journalistic routines of medical coverage; major changes to medical reporting during the epidemic; journalists' judgments on information-seeking as well as on angle and source selection while facing scientific and political uncertainty; journalists' reactions to criticism of news media performance during the SARS coverage; and what journalists learned about the news covering process from their experiences during the SARS epidemic.

Introduction: SARS outbreak and the news media in Taiwan

SARS took countries such as China, Hong Kong, Vietnam, Singapore, Canada, the US, and Taiwan by storm in early 2003. As early as mid-November 2002, there were already cases of pneumonia-like disease in China's Guangdong province. Aided by modern air travel, the local outbreak spread throughout the region in a matter of a few weeks. On 12 March 2003, the World Health Organization (WHO) issued a global alert on the outbreak of SARS (Koh, Plant, & Lee 2003). As Snodgrass (2003) indicates, in an era edgy with fears of world terrorism, SARS caused 17 nations to collaborate on anti-viral measures at borders, airports, hotels, hospitals, and on urban streets.

---

* An earlier version of this chapter was presented at the 54th Annual Conference of the International Communication Association, New Orleans, USA, 29 May 2004.

Due to frequent cross-straits travel between China and Taiwan via Hong Kong, the first SARS case in Taiwan appeared in late February, when a Taiwanese businessman who had been infected in Guangdong returned to Taiwan. By mid-April, although there had been sporadic cases of SARS in people returning from China, the health authorities stated that Taiwan still maintained a spotless record of "three zeros": zero deaths, zero community transmissions, and zero cases of Taiwanese taking the disease abroad. Because of this, WHO classified Taiwan as an "area with limited local transmission" (Chen, Chien, & Yang 2003). The health authorities remained in a state of blissful optimism, but it did not last long. On 22 April, several cases were discovered at Hoping Hospital in Taipei. On 24 April, the hospital was sealed off by the government after a series of mistakes led to a 'cluster' of SARS transmissions. The outbreak and the accompanying public panic then spread throughout Taiwan.

In Taiwan, SARS not only affected medical, social and economic areas, but also damaged the news media's image for accurate information dissemination and timely social integration. According to a survey conducted on 2 May 2003 by the Taiwanese Broadcasting Developing Fund, nearly 40% of the sample were not satisfied with SARS news coverage. Of those who were dissatisfied, 65% considered the SARS coverage too sensational, 29% thought it too negative, 17% believed the news media had failed to provide necessary information, and 16% mentioned that there were too many inaccurate reports (Lin 2003). Similarly, a study of public opinion on SARS in Taiwan and Hong Kong conducted in late May by the Academia Sinica, found that 44.4% of the Taiwanese sample attributed the perceived seriousness of the disease to the sensationalism of the news, but only 18.6% of the Hong Kong sample did so (Chu, Y. Chang., L. Chang, Lin, & C. Chang 2003).

Beyond the initial critical period, the news media continued to be the major source from which the public obtained information on SARS; but a surprisingly high proportion of Taiwanese were critical of the role the media had played at the peak of the outbreak. Such strong criticism emboldened intellectuals to write to media forums calling for more effort to improve the medical and social conditions of people in the lower social strata (Yang 2003). Discontent over the media performance even triggered various groups – such as medical workers, SARS patients, scholars, and local non-profit organizations – to disseminate SARS information on their own or to comment on SARS-related news reports by way of emails and websites (Lu 2004). There seemed to be a consensus amongst the public that SARS-related news reports had done little more than to label and frighten people.

These public reactions were supported by various news analyses in Taiwan. For example, the Foundation for the Advancement of Media Excellence (FAME), a local media watch organization, conducted a content analysis of SARS coverage in seven Taiwanese newspapers from March to May 2003. The study identified three types of poor news performance: false reports, sensational and exaggerated news, and violation of SARS patients' human rights (Lu 2004). Other studies found that political rather than medical and scientific forces dominated the framing of the SARS news discourse (Yang 2003), and that marginal social groups such as the homeless, working class (e.g., Liu 2004), and foreign laborers (e.g., Lin & Chen 2003) were stigmatized in the local news. Judging from the content of the Taiwanese SARS stories, the skepticism and criticism from the public did have some grounds.

Although most local voices in Taiwan focused on the news media's failure to fulfill their social responsibility, few analyzed the underlying factors that hindered the media from meeting the public needs in risk communication. It seemed that for an emerging infectious disease such as SARS, various forces involved in the interactions between the government, society, and the news media could lead the news production process away from risk control. This study does not examine all of the intertwined factors and relationships mentioned above. Rather, by examining the perceptions and experiences of medical journalists in covering SARS, the study explores why SARS reality was constructed in the Taiwanese media in the way it was.

Reporting health risks

A brief review of the features of health risk coverage and medical journalism will help provide a conceptual framework for the present study, although it should be noted that 'context' may play a critical role in determining how health risks are represented. Addressing the issue of communicating health risks to the public, Freimuth, Linnan and Potter (2000) indicated that public health officials often leave it to the news media to translate scientific and medical information for the lay person. Taiwan is no exception. On a more general level, research has shown that news media are important sources of health information for both individuals (Freimuth, Greenberg, DeWitt, & Romano 1984; Simpkins & Brenner 1984; Wallack 1990) and policy makers (Weiss 1974). Due to their prevalence in modern society, the news media sometimes have a stronger effect on public cognition, attitudes and preventive behavior than do more formal media campaigns. For example, news stories can deliver information on disease prevention in a more in-depth way than brief (paid or free) disease prevention messages (Freimuth, Linnan & Potter 2000). For those who have no direct contact with the disease or its sufferers, awareness of the disease is mostly media related.

Still, news media can serve both positive and negative functions in surveillance and social integration. Singer and Endreny (1993) surveyed a wide range of print and electronic media, looking at how various hazards were presented to the public, including communicable diseases. They argued that the accuracy and amount of information received from the environment, and perceptions of risk shaped by the media, may contribute to misguided individual and public choices for action and prevention.

Indeed, health risk coverage is shaped by the same constraints as other types of news stories. In addition to the commonly accepted news values of timeliness, proximity, consequence, human interest, conflict, prominence, and unusualness, Meyer (1990) argued that there are less visible constraints that also need to be taken into account: inoffensiveness, the window of credibility, fitting existing constructs, and being packable into daily bites. Health risk coverage can also be affected by market and political forces, as well as the difficulties journalists face in interpreting complicated health facts (Klaidman 1990; McCargo 2003; Meyer 1990; Stuyck 1990). Levi (2000) summarized ten types of "pitfalls" that are often encountered in medical journalism. Of these the following six will be helpful in understanding the controversy of the SARS coverage in Taiwan: reducing reporting to quoting; treating specialists as generalists; being misled by number games; depending on anecdotal evidence; mistaking risk factors for diseases; and misjudging risks.[1]

From the foregoing, intriguing questions arise: To what extent was SARS news in Taiwan a reflection of typical health risk coverage as outlined above? To what extent was SARS reporting affected by features that were specific to the journalistic routines and social contexts in Taiwan? What implications can be drawn from the experiences of medical journalists in SARS reports for future coverage of other emerging diseases?

Method: Qualitative interviews with medical journalists

This study focuses on how medical journalists made sense of their experiences of SARS reporting and of the structures of their journalistic routines. In other words, the focus is on processes rather than outcomes or products of the SARS coverage in Taiwan. To meet these assumptions (Creswell 1994; Merriam 1988),

---

1. The other four types of pitfalls mentioned by Levi (2000), which are more helpful in interpreting reporting of the development of medical science, are confusing science fiction with scientific facts; failing to question findings about a treatment's effects; extrapolating from research to clinical practice; and hyping a study's clinical implications.

a qualitative research design with in-depth semi-structured interviews was used to obtain information that could not be gained by observation (Berger 2000) or a content analysis of the news alone. Recruitment of journalists for the interviews was based on three criteria: working for the mainstream news media in Taiwan; having reported SARS extensively from April to June 2003; and having substantial experience in medical reporting.

The first step was to decide on the news media to be studied. The print media included the three most widely circulated newspapers – *China Times* (CT), *United Daily News* (UDN) and *Liberty Times* (LT) – and one newspaper with a specialized medical page for health professionals, *Min Seng Daily* (MSD). From the electronic media, two wireless network television stations – *China Television* (CTV) and *Chinese Television Service* (CTS) – were chosen, as was the highest rating cable news channel, *TVBS News*. Of these media organizations, the ownership of the *Liberty Times* is known for its pro-ruling party (Democratic Progressive Party or DPP) stand; a major shareholding of *Chinese Television Service* belongs to the ministries of Education and Defense; the *China Times, United Daily News* and *Min Seng Daily* are aligned with opposition parties – the Kuomintang (KMT) and the People First Party or (PFP). *China Television* is owned by the major opposition party, the KMT. The effects of political forces on media ownership will be discussed when the conflicts reflected in the SARS-related coverage are examined.

A databank news search was then conducted for medical journalists from the selected news media who matched the three criteria. After excluding those who were unavailable at the time of the study, eight in-depth interviews were conducted between 24 June and 21 July 2003. The interviews averaged from two to four hours in length. The abbreviated names of the journalists, the news media with which they were affiliated, their background and professional experiences, and interview dates are listed in Table 1. Coincidentally, the interviewees were all female, which roughly reflects the gender structure of medical journalists in Taiwan. Interviews were conducted with two journalists from the *Liberty Times* because, after completing the first interview with BL, a follow-up was needed with someone who had a different perspective.

During each interview, a list of general topics was provided to help uncover the interviewee's perspective. Generally, each interviewee's framing and structuring of responses was respected (Marshall & Rossman 1989). Probes were used whenever necessary. Five broad issues were explored: (a) journalistic routines of medical coverage; (b) major changes of medical reporting during the epidemic; (c) journalists' judgments on information-seeking, story angle, and source selection while facing scientific and political uncertainty; (d) journalists' reactions to criticism (e.g., from government, academics, public and medical professionals) of news media performance during the SARS coverage; and (e) journalists'

Table 1. Medical journalists interviewed in the study

Name of journalist	News media	Background/professional experience	Date of interview
XW	United Daily News (UDN)	Majored in nursing and mass communication; 7 years of medical reporting	21 June 2003
BL	Liberty Times (LT)	Majored in mass communication; 12 years of medical reporting	21 June 2003
LC	China Times (CT)	Majored in economics and journalism; 9 years of medical reporting	24 June 2003
HY	China Television News (CTV)	Majored in journalism; 6 years of medical reporting	27 June 2003
WW	TVBS News (TVBS)	Majored in mass communication; 5 years of medical reporting	27 June 2003
CH	Min Seng Daily (MSD)	Majored in Chinese literature; 5 years of medical reporting	7 July 2003
YP	Chinese Television Service (CTS)	Majored in philosophy and journalism; 5 years of medical reporting	8 July 2003
FC	Liberty Times (LT)	Majored in mass communication and social medicine; 5 years of medical reporting	24 July 2003

experiences learned from and problems faced, in the news covering process. To help interviewees address these issues more efficiently, major SARS events were used as prompts during the interviews. These key events will be discussed together with the analysis in the next section.

Analysis: Journalists' interpretations of SARS coverage

The eight interviews were first transcribed literally, and then their content was re-grouped according to the five issues outlined above. The important findings generated from the interviews are summarized in the five sections below, which are supplemented with representative quotations from individual journalists. SARS events and news stories are introduced as background information whenever necessary.

Journalistic routines of medical coverage

On average, print media were staffed with seven to nine medical reporters. Medical journalists at the television stations were much fewer than their newspaper counterparts. For example, there was only one journalist at CTS and three at

TVBS assigned to health coverage, together with other issues categorized into 'life' or 'living'. Medical reporters at the *Liberty Times* (LT) were also required to write soft and human-interest health tips or columns for the health page. To compete with the arrival in Taiwan's news market of *Apple Daily*, a Hong Kong-based tabloid, health reporting within the *United Daily News* (UDN) had shifted focus from all straight news to more human interest stories in early March 2003. A medical reporting team was formed, with most of the team considered novices in medical coverage.

Generally, medical reporting has not been highly valued by Taiwanese news media. The turnover rates of medical reporters are quite high, although some news media such as the *China Times* (CT) claimed that they would not employ novices to report health and medicine. All interviewees indicated that hospitals and health authorities (e.g., Department of Health, Center for Disease Control) were their major news sources. Assignments for the print media reporters were decided by grouping major hospitals, medical centers and adjacent health administrations together to be covered by the same reporter. *Min Seng Daily* (MSD), a newspaper having an entire health page targeted at health professionals, appeared to be the only news medium in which medical journalists were involved in the news-editing process. That is, MSD reporters write both the stories and the headlines. Differences between the journalistic routines of the news media did affect how SARS stories were presented, a point that will be returned to later.

Major changes of medical reporting during SARS

The outbreak of SARS in Taiwan caused the news media to reshuffle their news assignments due to a huge demand in coverage.[2] The *Min Seng Daily* was the lone exception. According to the other journalists, many non-health reporters were re-assigned to support the SARS beats. For example, YP at CTS indicated that two-thirds of all reporters in her news department were devoted to SARS coverage, regardless of the original assignments that they were responsible for. Working for the print medium, XW (UDN) also mentioned that as many as 10 reporters from other beats came to assist in SARS coverage during the peak of the epidemic. As reporting of SARS involved judgment on scientific uncertainties or risks, whether journalists unfamiliar with medical coverage could handle their beats appropriately was a question for concern.

---

2. As many non-medical reporters were assigned to cover SARS on an unscheduled and un-planned basis within most news organizations, information regarding the exact number of total journalists involved in SARS coverage is unavailable.

This concern seemed to be further complicated by the reporters' shift from relying on one expert source to relying on multiple sources, which was another major change of medical reporting during SARS. Several journalists indicated that they had started to lose confidence in official sources, which were too slow in reacting to breaking events and sometimes released incomplete or inaccurate information. Reliance on core expert sources had been considered the norm during the journalists' previous routine medical coverage. However, some expert sources, probably due to their resistance to being misquoted or being treated as scientist-know-all generalists, became cautious about expressing opinions during the epidemic. To meet their deadlines, as revealed by XW (UDN), reporters were forced to look for alternative sources, who may have been less credible but were more willing to talk to the press. Consequently, the chances of news stories being published with inaccurate, exaggerated or unconfirmed information became much higher.

The following instance illustrates the problem caused by the participation of non-medical reporters, not-so-credible sources, or a combination of both in the SARS reporting. At the early stage of the outbreak, there was a prevailing fear of becoming the next mass transportation victim to be infected by SARS, as had previously happened to passengers on trains and inter-city buses. Various socially disadvantaged groups were also labeled as carriers of the virus. The homeless were constructed in the news as the "dead corner" in battling "the war on SARS." Foreign care-givers in the hospitals, foreign domestic maids, and illegal immigrants were targeted as "walking carriers" or "moving carriers" who "invisibly" transmitted the disease to the general public (Lin & Chen 2003; Liu 2004; Yang 2003).

The presentation of SARS news, however, changed again after the Government Information Office (GIO), the state institution in charge of licensing Taiwan's broadcast media, decided to become involved. All three television news reporters felt the change in their news production and editing processes, particularly in handling pictures and cuts. As YP at CTS put it, "the GIO invited managers of the news departments from all television stations over for communication. After this morality lesson, our newsroom policy changed."

Judgment-making on uncertainty

Another issue in the study concerned medical journalists' judgments on information seeking, story angle, and source selection amidst scientific and political uncertainty. At the beginning of the SARS epidemic, there were divergent theories on how the virus spread. The market responded to this sudden virus of uncertain origin and unknown cure with all kinds of prescriptions and formulas that were rumored to prevent SARS. Things like bee propolis, lingzhi fungus, isatis root, and multi-vitamins were all said to increase immunity (Lee 2003). When the outbreak first occurred in Taipei's Hoping Hospital, the public trust in the government's ability to control the SARS virus effectively faded. Experts were divided over the real efficacy of various protective devices against SARS. With great uncertainty surrounding the epidemic, questions were raised about the shutting down of all business and public venues and all commercial activities, as well as the mandatory wearing of protective masks in public places. Therefore, efforts to clarify uncertainties were left to the news media.

Most journalists admitted that decision-making of this kind was very difficult. For example, YP (CTS), a broadcast reporter who seemed confident in voicing her decision-making process, indicated that when facing conflicting information from the health and medical authorities, she would just select those that she herself trusted. Moreover, YP and the other two television reporters interviewed, CH at TVBS and HY at China Television, also emphasized that the key to a good television news story was 'pictures', and that this dominated their decision-making on sources.

BL (LT), who had 12 years of medical reporting experience, indicated that she trusted scholars most. However, LC (CT), who had nine years of experience, argued that medical reporting should be more thoughtful. "You cannot simply use your first impression in reporting SARS." This is indeed true when journalists confronted health officials who released conflicting information many times a day. "You get smarter with time," said FC (LT), who was quite outspoken about the unprofessional performances of several top health officials. CH (MSD) would exhaust all useful sources for an uncertain issue, but she also indicated that easing public anxiety was more important. Thus, for example, even though she doubted the real effectiveness of masks against the virus, she would still quote sources who promoted mask wearing in public.

Most reporters admitted that they were reluctant to "bother" the same sources all of the time, but as XW (UDN) put it, "we have no other choices. Only a few people know about SARS. We need reliable and credible sources to pass useful information to the public." However, as discussed earlier, many reporters were forced to look for new sources as the journalistic routine of reliance on some core sources was no longer feasible. Overall, there were quite a variety of styles amongst the medical journalists, although some of the facts that the journalists revealed in retrospect appeared defensive and were thus questionable.

Furthermore, when asked whether they had checked for further information on international websites, such as that of the WHO or those of other countries that were struck by SARS, almost all of the journalists indicated that they were working under time pressure. Taiwan's Center for Disease Control website seemed to be their major source of SARS information on the Internet. In fact, most of journalists were even surprised at being asked such a question, as though the issue had never occurred to them.

Judging from the foregoing, to get the stories reported on time and meet deadlines was still the journalists' top priority during the SARS crisis. Time pressure increased the risk of not covering the epidemic precisely. The journalists had written all sorts of stories with both accurate and inaccurate information. They had also submitted news reports to the editing staff with confirmed and unconfirmed information. It was thus left to the news editors to determine what should be published. In this regard, the kind of caution normally required in medical reporting seemed to give way to concern over competition amongst the media. This phenomenon will be addressed in more detail in the next section.

Reactions to criticism of news media performance

There has been strong criticism in Taiwanese society of the news media's performance during the SARS coverage, including from the government, academics, public, and medical professionals. Hence, it is pertinent to ask whether it is possible to distinguish between the negative effect of the news media's poor performance and that generated by other forces, such as the government and the public. Some journalists admitted that the news media were indeed too sloppy and sensational in SARS reporting; others, however, pointed out that the news coverage had simply exposed problems in government and society that had been there for a long time.

To elaborate the problems of the latter, even the most senior health official of the Center for Disease Control indicated that "the weakness of disease control in Taiwan was totally revealed" (Su 2003). As indicated by several of the interviewees, for two months after the SARS epidemic had begun, the Department of Health had not established fixed procedures for handling suspected cases. The hospitals did not necessarily have adequate resources to defend against the virus. Some health care professionals had nothing more useful than raincoats to wear when approaching infectious SARS patients, which suggested that the government was not well prepared and had no experience in dealing with an outbreak of this magnitude.[3] The

---

3. Senior health officials contended that Taiwan had well-trained medical personnel and excellent facilities, but because it was not able to get advice and practical support from the WHO in a timely manner – such as on preventing hospital transmission and implementing in-hospital prevention measures – much energy was misspent and the holes created by mistakes were not plugged. Vietnam, in contrast, had far fewer resources, but received a great deal of WHO help and was able to rapidly control the spread of the virus (Lee 2003).

public also lacked awareness and self-discipline. These are just some of the reasons for the magnification of the negative effect of SARS on society.

Coming back to the criticisms of news coverage of SARS, the interviewees provided various interpretations of why there had been problems of serious false reports, sensational and exaggerated news, and violations of SARS patients' human rights. Of course, when considering such criticisms it should be kept in mind that it sometimes would have been difficult to separate media responsibility from institutional responsibility in detecting the source of any 'flaws' in the news content.

(1) False and sensational reports
The accuracy of information and the perceptions of risk shaped by the media contributed to misguided individual and public choices for action and prevention during the SARS outbreak. FC (LT) indicated that she had made mistakes in her SARS stories because she did not double check with various sources. CH (MSD) also recalled one major mistake she made by asking the wrong sources for reporting a conflicting event involving SARS patient transfer. She, however, complained that people tended to subject press performance to great scrutiny during the SARS epidemic. HW (UDN) admitted that sometimes she simply did not know how to handle tons of SARS-related information she received every day. Reflecting on journalists' performances, she explained that medical reporters needed to have more professional knowledge to clarify certain scientific facts and figures for the public, and not just introduce basic information about the epidemic, as released by the government.

Regardless of the reasons given by the journalists, a lack of awareness about the seriousness of the SARS epidemic and the journalists' lack of sufficient medical knowledge tended to account for some of the criticisms raised. Most of the time, however, sensational and false SARS-related reports resulted largely from the interplay between individual journalists and institutional (both the news media and the government) forces.

The *United Daily's* inaccurate report on water infection in the Huachang Public Housing Project serves as a good example. In early May, when it appeared that the epidemic had been brought more or less under control in Taipei City, there was a wave of cases of SARS in individuals with no known history of contact with infected persons. On 10 May, an elderly person living alone in an apartment in the Huachang Public Housing Project was discovered to have passed away at home several days previously, and two women living in neighboring apartments (one of whom died shortly thereafter) were apparently infected. The entire community was quickly sealed off, with more than 700 persons subjected to compulsory quarantine, making this the first community in Taiwan to be sealed as a result of a SARS outbreak. On the day that Huachang was sealed off, the World Health

Organization listed Taipei, along with Beijing, Guangdong, Shan'xi and Hong Kong, as an area of high incidence of SARS transmission.

Even though the Huachang community was sealed off, it was still uncertain whether there had been an infection of the water system or shared public facilities. Nevertheless, the news media, including the *Liberty Times, United Daily News* and *China Times,* used language which either implied that the community was infected or hinted at who the "super spreader" was without citing appropriate sources. UDN even used "Virus-loaded Water, Wanhua Community Infection Breaks Out" as the headline for the front-page story on 10 May. An investigation later showed that there had been no infection of the water system, and the neighborhood was released from quarantine.

According to XW (UDN), the *United Daily* story was written by a political reporter assisting on the SARS beat. The story on Huachang was framed as a political struggle between DPP state health officials and the KMT Taipei City Government. Information provided by a Taipei City Government spokesperson, who was more familiar with political than health matters, was used to challenge the central government's ability to control the community infection. This somehow echoed UDN's long-term, underlying political ideology, which was further reflected in how the editor handled stories and headlines. A similar example can be found in UDN's framing of the SARS-related policies of the then Minister of the Department of Health and loyal DPP supporter, Shiing-Jer Twu. In the news headlines, Twu's political dimension seemed to be more negatively presented than other aspects of his policy-making.

Although the pro-oppositional party UDN did not bother to suppress its politically tinted stand in covering the Huachang event, other news media were more cautious. LC (CT), also working for a pro-oppositional party news organization, did not hide her derision of the then Minister Twu when addressing his professionalism and personality. LC also did not appreciate the public relations skills that Twu had frequently used on the reporters. Nevertheless, she insisted on professional medical reporting and strongly opposed politicizing SARS coverage. When LC found that the stories she wrote were edited with sensational or faulty headlines, she would communicate with the editors or her superiors to ask for corrections.

In fact, most journalists agreed that the political struggle between the ruling central government and the opposition-led Taipei City Government had in some way deterred the efficient control of SARS. For instance, XW (UDN) did not necessarily agree with what her news organization had been doing in highlighting the political tone of the SARS-related stories, particularly linking fact-based stories that she had written with politicized headlines. However, when asked whether she had expressed her opinions to the editor, she replied that there did not seem to be a communication channel through which she could do that.

Aside from the problems resulting from the news media's underlying political ideology, variations of newsroom policy within the news organizations, and individual differences in journalists' reactions to the inaccurate reports, false SARS information did occasionally come from news sources, be they central or local governments. As LC (CT) mentioned, "health authorities were giving confusing or even false information and sometimes it was corrected by the reporters during the press conferences." XW (UDN) said that "fighting an epidemic is much like fighting a war . . . the magnitude of the SARS coverage was much broader than we expected. We all could not help but make mistakes." Working for a pro-ruling party press, BL (LT) argued that the news media had the responsibility to help the health authorities control the epidemic, echoing her news organization's support for the state health authority.

(2) Sensationalism and the violation of human rights

During the initial stage of the SARS outbreak, words loaded with fear appeal such as "virus airplane," "dangerous airplane" and "you are flying with patients with horrible pneumonia" were used quite often in the news media (Liu 2004). Rumors, descriptions of unconfirmed suspected cases, and the use of criminal metaphors were also common in the related stories. News coverage like this was particularly serious when the Hoping Hospital in Taipei was hurriedly sealed off in late April,[4] followed by the closing of other hospitals around Taiwan.

From 25 April, virtually every day there were new cases of medical staff and patients at Hoping showing high fever, and with the hospital failing to take timely measures to more strictly isolate affected persons, the virus spread quickly and could not be contained (Lee 2003). In fact, according to Taiwan's CDC (2003), about 90% of SARS cases in Taiwan were the result of hospital transmission. In late April, the SARS infection rate for medical personnel reached 32%. With regards to this issue, the interviewees all indicated that tracing infected cases was the top priority of their coverage. Hence, one patient, a Ms. Tsao, was described as "super spreader." Headlines such as "where does she live?" and "the fall of Hoping Hospital,

---

4. Early in April, a woman from Taipei named Tsao went to southern Taiwan to visit her mother-in-law, who was in hospital there. On her return north, she became infected by SARS, probably a result of being in the same rail car as an infected individual from the Amoy Gardens housing project in Hong Kong (where dozens of people had come down with the disease). Ms Tsao went to the Hoping Hospital, and although the hospital was on the lookout for possible cases and immediately transferred her to a better equipped teaching hospital, in the brief time that she had spent in Hoping – less than one hour – her presence set off a chain reaction with explosive results.

epidemic out of control" were used frequently. Instead of discussing what caused SARS, people, especially SARS patients, were described as being responsible for the outbreak. The news media even legitimized their voyeurism in spying on those who were quarantined, which drew criticism as a violation of human rights.

LC (CT) provided two perspectives on this matter. First, she mentioned that spokespersons of the health authorities sometimes did not perform their roles well: that is, they were not tight-lipped about the privacy of the patients. They would unintentionally reveal patient information in private to those journalists with whom they were more familiar. That information then became news headlines in some media. Secondly, the health authorities did tell journalists to protect patients' privacy. At the beginning, there was a consensus amongst most journalists that the identity of patients should be protected. Nevertheless, once one publication exposed the names, the others followed. As XW (UDN) put it, reporters at the *United Daily* never intruded on patients' privacy, unless reporters of other news organizations had done so first.

The news media were also criticized for informing their readers of where SARS patients lived, which caused discrimination from neighbors and whole communities. In defending her news organization, YP (CTS) argued that it was *Next Magazine*, a Hong Kong-based tabloid, which revealed the names first. LC (CT) also said that the news media sometimes obtained most information, especially names, from the hospitals, which did not have tight control over patient information at the beginning of the epidemic. Later, like detectives, reporters tried to link information gained from various sources together to compile a profile of the cases. FC (LT) indicated that they sometimes did not really know where to draw the line, especially when the reporter found that the cases could be very good stories. Most interviewees mentioned that once the patient appeared in the stories often, anonymity or fake names would simply confuse readers when they wanted to relate new stories to previous events.

Nevertheless, it seemed that some of the interviewees were trying to avoid taking responsibility for public criticism. Although it was obvious that the institutional sources, such as the government officials and the hospital staff, were careless in handling issues of patients' privacy rights, the news media did not fully practice the power of the fourth estate. On the contrary, most of the news media (or journalists in particular) simply performed as coercive apparatuses in magnifying the institutional flaws that were already apparent. Amongst all of the pitfalls faced by the medical journalists, this should have been the most avoidable.

Experience gained

For good or bad, what did the journalists learn from their involvement in SARS news reporting? All of the interviewees indicated that they had worked over-time and had been devoted to covering SARS during the peak of the epidemic. As they may have had direct contact with families of SARS patients and health profession-als who had contact with the patients, some interviewees mentioned that they had to stay in hotels, and were not allowed to go back to the news organizations. In other words, the medical reporters thought they were also discriminated against. Therefore, criticism from the government, the public, and academia about their performance hurt their feelings quite a bit. Regardless of this, most interviewees considered their involvement in SARS reporting, especially in reporting the seal-ing off of Hoping Hospital, to be the most unforgettable work experience they had ever had.

Some medical journalists who were more reflective considered themselves to have been part of the battle against SARS. As LC (CT) put it, "not only did I search the information for the public, but I also did that for myself." YP (CTS) said that reporting SARS was like a news war, and that journalists were placed in a very special and important position. The most difficult part was to double check or confirm facts under time pressure, especially for television news. CH (MSD), however, argued that the news confirmation process during SARS was actually similar to what medical journalists were doing at normal times. The only differ-ence was that people paid more attention to the accuracy of SARS information. In retrospect, XW (UDN) felt that a medical reporter needs more professional knowledge to cover health or disease control, not only knowledge just in intro-ducing basic facts to the public, but also in how to clarify scientific facts more efficiently. In this regard, XW gave one of the very few interviewees' accounts that were characterized more by reflexivity than reminiscence of heroic deeds in the SARS reporting battle.

Summary and implications

The widespread SARS epidemic enveloped the entire island of Taiwan in a mist of anxiety and tragedy for a few months. Problems that had long been lurking were exposed. Various sectors of society, including the government, health care ser-vices, general public and, of course, the news media, all came to reconsider how their relationships with one another would affect how health risks were perceived, communicated, and handled. Development into a society of diverse cultures en-abled Taiwanese people to be critical of news media performance (Chang 2004).

It also led the media to have less trust in the establishment, and thus become more cynical about the government's performance.

Overall, the findings presented in this chapter help to build an exploratory understanding of how and why SARS reality was constructed in the Taiwanese media. The foregoing analysis showed that SARS reporting in Taiwan did in some way reflect typical health risk coverage as outlined in the relevant communication literature. In addition to an emphasis on the features of news values such as proximity, consequence, human interest, conflict, and unusualness (Meyer 1990), the SARS coverage was affected by market and political forces, as well as journalists' difficulties in interpreting complicated health facts (Klaidman 1990; Meyer 1990; Stuyck 1990; Wilkins 2005).

The problems found in the SARS coverage also resonated with the pitfalls pointed out by Levi (2000). For instance, journalists tended to overuse quotes from expert sources, sometimes with stories that were simply compiled from various quotes. This became a vicious circle: expert sources became resistant to the unprofessional interviews, which forced journalists to resort to sources who were less credible but more willing to be interviewed, and reduced the quality of news reporting. The reliance of journalists on anecdotal evidence and mistaking marginalized people as high-risk groups, or even worse, misjudging risks for the infectious disease, also contributed to unnecessary public panic and stigmatization.

Moreover, SARS reporting was affected by features that were specific to individual journalists, journalistic routines and social/political contexts in Taiwan. On a more micro-level, the failure of journalists to take the SARS epidemic seriously was due partly to their lack of sufficient medical knowledge. The interviews revealed that journalists' sensitivity to and perception of the issue made a difference to their reporting. Some journalists valued their experiences in participating in the SARS coverage, but others did not seem to notice that the reporting of the SARS outbreak needed to be different from their routine health coverage.

Journalists' perceptions of the uniqueness of the SARS coverage were further affected by the attitudes and decision-making styles of their superiors. The print media journalists that were interviewed tended to be more reflective than their electronic media counterparts. In addition, although experience and training were important, how the journalists handled information about uncertainty and reacted to the distortion of their stories in the newsroom, as well as their relationships with various news sources, determined their sense of empowerment and self importance in covering the emerging disease.

Judging from the foregoing, it appears critical to strengthen the professional knowledge of journalists and their ability to adapt to crisis reporting. This can be done by more in-service training within news organizations or by workshops sponsored by non-media professional organizations. Training of this type is particularly important to the current medical reporting because increasing numbers of novices have recently joined the medical reporting teams in the news organizations.

The analysis also found that a seemingly high news or market value of sensational information came to dominate journalists' judgments about rights or privacy matters. This raises questions about the criteria of news worthiness in times of risk control or even crisis. Does the presumed market value of sensationalism really meet the needs of the public in risk control, or is it the other way around? Perhaps more importantly, news media need to reconsider their standard operating procedures for the news production process. An interface for better communication between the reporters and the editing staff must also be devised. This is particularly crucial when news assignments are reshuffled in times of crisis. These measures should minimize the unnecessary influences of political ideology in the representation and interpretation of the health risk issues or events.

Lastly, the analysis showed that news coverage in Taiwan cannot avoid being affected by market and political forces. Therefore, instead of suggesting that news media play the so-called 'objective' role in reporting issues or events, it is more important for the Taiwanese news media to value the increasing impact of globalization, including the widespread phenomenon of emerging infectious diseases. In addition to producing more in-depth and less sensational health risk reports, the news media may well seriously consider reframing their stories in a less provincial manner. By doing so, they will be able to empower their reporting and editing staff with more adequate knowledge, skills and perceptions to meet the growing risk or crisis coverage demands that have been discussed in this chapter.

References

Berger, A. A. (2000). *Media and communication research methods: An introduction to qualitative and quantitative approaches.* Thousand Oaks, CA: Sage.

Carmichael, M. (2003, May 5). Economies on empty. *Newsweek*, p. 18.

Center for Disease Control, Taiwan. (2003). *Memoir of Severe Acute Respiratory Syndrome control in Taiwan.* Taipei: Center for Disease Control.

Chang, C. (2004). *A risk reporting analysis on SARS reports from foreign correspondents based in China and reports from Taiwanese local media.* Paper presented at the annual conference of Chinese Communication Association. Macao, China.

Chen, C., Chien, Y., & Yang, H. (2003). Epidemiology and control of Severe Acute Respiratory Syndrome (SARS) outbreak in Taiwan. In T. Koh, A. Plant, & E. H. Lee (Eds.), *The new global threat: Severe Acute Respiratory Syndrome and its impacts* (pp. 301–313). Singapore: World Scientific.

Chu, H., Chang, Y., Chang, L., Lin, F., & Chang, C. (2003). A survey report on the social trends during SARS epidemic. In M. Lai (Ed.), *SARS in spring, 2003: A review of the science, society and culture of SARS epidemic* (pp. 149–194). Taipei: Linking Publisher.

Creswell, J. W. (1994). *Research design: Qualitative & quantitative approaches*. Thousand Oaks, CA: Sage.

Freimuth, V. S., Linnan, H. W., & Potter, P. (2000). Communicating the threat of emerging infections to the public. *Emerging Infectious Diseases, 6*, 337–347.

Freimuth, V. S., Greenberg, R. H., DeWitt, J., & Romano, R. M. (1984). Covering cancer: Newspapers and the public interest. *Journal of Communication, 34*(1), 62–73.

Klaidman, S. (1990). Roles and responsibilities of journalists. In C. Atkin & L. Wallack (Eds.), *Mass communication and public health* (pp. 60–70). Newbury Park, CA: Sage.

Koh, T., Plant, A., & Lee, E. H. (2003). WHO: At the forefront of combating SARS. In T. Koh, A. Plant, & E. H. Lee (Eds.), *The new global threat: Severe Acute Respiratory Syndrome and its impacts* (pp. 3–13). Singapore: World Scientific.

Lee, L. (2003, June). SARS wars: Taiwan fights a battle it cannot afford to lose. *Sinorama, 28*(6), 6–17.

Leung, P. C. (2003). Editorial. In P. C. Leung & E. E. Ooi (Eds.), *SARS war: Combating the disease* (pp. 1–9). Singapore: World Scientific.

Levi, R. (2001). *Medical journalism: Exposing fact, fiction, fraud*. Ames: Iowa State University Press.

Lin, Y. (2003). Qualitative analyses of SARS news reports by the domestic press: The cases of Huachang public housing complex quarantine and the alleged SOS letter in a bottle from Mackay Memorial Hospital. *Thought and Words: Journal of the Humanities and Social Science, 41*(4), 71–110.

Lin, Y., & Chen, B. (2003, November). *Representation of and audience reactions to foreign laborers in the SARS news*. Paper presented at the Conference on Globalization and News Reports. Taipei, Taiwan.

Liu, C. (2004). *From invisible to visible: Representation of others in SARS news coverage*. Unpublished master's thesis. National Chengchi University, Taiwan.

Lu, S. (2004, January*). Media advocacy and social mobilization during SARS epidemic*. Conference on SARS and Sustainable Development. Taipei, Taiwan.

Marshall, C., & Rossman, G. B. (1989). *Designing qualitative research*. Thousand Oaks, CA: Sage.

McCargo, D. (2003). *Media and politics in Pacific Asia*. London and New York: Routledge Curzon.

Merriam, S. B. (1988). *Case study research in education: A qualitative approach*. San Francisco: Jossey-Bass.

Meyer, P. (1990). News media responsiveness to public health. In C. Atkin & L. Wallack (Eds.), *Mass communication and public health* (pp. 52–59). London: Sage.

Simpkins, J. D., & Brenner, D. J. (1984). Mass media communication and health. In B. Dervin & M. J. Voigt (Eds.), *Progress in communication sciences* (pp. 275–297). Norwood, NJ: Ablex.

Singer, E., & Endreny, P. M. (1993). *Reporting on risk: How the mass media portray accidents, diseases, disasters and other hazards*. New York: Russell Sage Foundation.

Snodgrass, M. E. (2003). *World epidemics: A cultural chronology of disease from prehistory to the era of SARS*. Jefferson, NC: McFarland.

Stuyck, S. C. (1990). Public health and the media: Unequal partners? In C. Atkins & L. Wallack (Eds.), *Mass communication and public health: Complexities and conflicts* (pp. 71–77). Newbury Park, CA: Sage.

Su, I. J. (2003). Foreword. *Memoir of Severe Acute Respiratory Syndrome control in Taiwan.* Taipei: Center for Disease Control, Taiwan.

Wallack, L. (1990). Mass media and health promotion: Promise, problem, and challenge. In C. Atkin & L. Wallack (Eds.), *Mass communication and public health* (pp. 41–50). Newbury Park, CA: Sage.

Weiss, C. H. (1974). What America's leaders read. *Public Opinion Quarterly, 38,* 1–21.

Wilkins, L. (2005). Plagues, pestilence and pathogens: The ethical implications of news reporting of a world health crisis. *Asian Journal of Communication, 15,* 247–254.

Yang, F. (2003). Class anxiety – "Chinese pneumonia" – the WHO as battlefield. In *Infectious: SARS in the world media,* Retrieved from http://www.opendemocracy.net/themes/article-8-1309.jsp#21.

Yang, S. (2003, November). *From medical to heroic discourse: Political power and media manipulation in the SARS news events.* Paper presented at the Conference on Globalization and News Reports. Taipei, Taiwan.

PART IV

Cross national constructions of SARS

CHAPTER 11

Newspaper coverage of the 2003 SARS outbreak

J. Brian Houston,[1] Wen-yu Chao[2] and Sandra Ragan[2]
[1]University of Oklahoma Health Sciences Center / [2]University of Oklahoma

SARS suddenly emerged in 2003 and became the first global health threat in the modern mass mediated era. A content analysis was undertaken to determine how the media in four different countries covered the SARS outbreak, in order to understand how the media construct a global health threat. Results indicate that the media relied on thematic treatments of SARS, most often utilizing a topic focused on statistical representations of the number of SARS deaths and victims. The media also focused on the isolation and quarantines imposed due to SARS. Other topics varied in frequency depending on how close or remote the media sources were to the SARS outbreak. Government entities were the most frequent sources of information in all coverage of the SARS outbreak.

On February 11, 2003, *The South China Morning Post* ran an article headlined: *Panic grips Guangdong as mystery pneumonia-like virus kills 6* (Ying & Lee 2003). This was the Hong Kong paper's first mention of the SARS outbreak that would eventually infect 8096 individuals worldwide – killing 774 of those infected (World Health Organization [WHO] 2004). SARS is a respiratory disease caused by a coronavirus, the same type of virus that causes the common cold (Center for Disease Control [CDC] 2003). However, unlike the common cold, SARS killed 9.6% of those reported to have contracted it, with mortality rates as high as 17% in Toronto and Hong Kong – two hot spots of the SARS outbreak (WHO 2004).

In Hong Kong, one of the hardest hit areas of the SARS outbreak, schools and hospitals were closed, entire apartment buildings that had housed SARS-infected individuals were quarantined, and many citizens wore surgical masks on city streets to protect themselves against exposure to the SARS virus (Bradsher 2003). Within a few months, SARS emerged from nonexistence to become a worldwide health crisis whose conclusion and implications for humanity were then unknown (Abraham 2007).

The age of mass mediated human existence has not seen the sudden emergence of a biological human threat equal to SARS. The uniqueness of the SARS outbreak provides an excellent opportunity to examine the role of the mass media in defining a new health crisis. As such, looking at mass media coverage of the SARS outbreak will add to the general literature on mass media constructions of health, as well as provide an account of how the mass media construct a new biological threat to the human race.

Media coverage of health issues

Understanding media coverage of health-related issues is important for two reasons. First, media depictions of health issues are key influences on how a disease or illness is understood within a culture. As Clarke (1992) writes, "intertwined with the experience of disease is the media's portrayal of disease. The media portrayal may affect the social relations, the self-images, the economic and political positions of persons with the disease, their loved ones and others" (p. 105). An example of the power of media constructions of disease is the way in which the AIDS epidemic was originally treated. Through specific media frames and metaphors, AIDS coverage created "risk groups" as opposed to risk behaviors, and, as a result, AIDS became a disease associated with a specific group of people rather than a disease that was communicable through specific behaviors (Bardhan 2002). The frame or metaphor utilized by the media to explain a disease forms the social schema by which individuals in a society understand both the disease and the individuals who are living with the disease (Lakoff & Johnson 2000).

Secondly, media coverage of health issues shapes the way individuals understand what should be done to prevent or treat a disease (Bardhan 2002). The relationship between the media and disease prevention and treatment is a natural one because communication is essential to any prevention effort, and the media are agents of mass communication (Rogers 2000). In fact, the media are understood to be a primary source of medical and health information – usually cited second only to an individual's doctor (Bractic & Greenberg 1979). The ability of the mass media to create a single message that reaches many people allows the media to educate audiences on how disease can be averted and prevented. Messages intended to increase prevention and treatment of illness must inform the population about what a disease is and which actions are necessary for treatment and prevention, and the message must motivate that audience to follow the prescriptive guidelines and take action against the disease (Freimuth, Edgar, & Hammond 1987; Freimuth, Hammond, Edgar, & Monahan 1990).

The idea that the media can inform and motivate the public to take specific action regarding health issues is related to the idea that the media act as an educator and have the responsibility to deliver information concerning social benefits and "socially beneficial ideas, behaviors or beliefs" (Winett & Wallack 1996, p. 173). This type of normative conception of the mass media draws heavily on the goals of social marketing, in which the purpose of messages are to advise, educate, and inform the audience about what can be done to make their lives better and safer (Flay & Burton 1990; Lefebvre & Flora 1988).

As a result of the importance of mediated coverage of health issues, media and health researchers have undertaken many studies focused on understanding how disease is constructed in the media and how specific media constructions of disease affect society. Another goal of researchers investigating mediated constructions of health issues is the hope that through this line of research specific normative guidelines will be identified that allow for the improvement of disease prevention and treatment within a population as a result of improved mediated coverage of that disease.

Research following the first line of investigation – i.e., attempts to understand how illness is constructed – includes Clarke's (1992) study on media coverage of cancer, heart disease, and AIDS. Clarke found that media constructions created an understanding that cancer was a disease that intruded into one's body leading to excruciating suffering and ultimately death. Cancer was also constructed as a disease that is preventable either through early checkups or lifestyle changes. As a result of this construction, cancer is understood to be, to an extent, the fault of the patient for not behaving differently. A much different media construction was used for a heart attack, which is "presented as an objective, morally neutral event that happens at one time and in a specific place to an individual who experiences a great deal of pain" (Clark, p. 115). Unlike cancer, heart disease is viewed optimistically as a treatable, recoverable event. Finally, AIDS is presented in the most negative terms of the three diseases in that "the person with AIDS is portrayed as a diseased person, as morally repugnant, hopelessly doomed, and isolated from potentially significant sources of emotional support such as lovers and family members" (Clarke, p. 117). In an effort similar to Clarke's, McAllister and Kitron (2003) compared press coverage of AIDS to Lyme disease, finding that coverage of Lyme disease had a lighter tone compared to stories focusing on AIDS and also finding that people associated with Lyme disease were portrayed more sympathetically than those associated with AIDS.

The second line of research involves studies that hope to improve normative communicative strategies for health communication. Examples of this line include Wellings' (1988) examination of the media content of AIDS, which found that as a result of the frames utilized by the media to explain the AIDS epidemic, people were confused as to what actions they should take in response to AIDS. Freimuth, Hammond, Edgar, and Monahan (1990) and Bardhan (2002) examined AIDS prevention campaigns executed through the media, identified types of messages used, and constructed guidelines to help future communicators create effective public health messages. Menashe and Siegel (1998) compared pro-tobacco to anti-tobacco frames used in the media in hopes of understanding why tobacco use remains pervasive within the United States in spite of the wealth of evidence pointing to tobacco's harmful health effects. Mebane, Temin, and Parvanta (2003) examined CDC and media coverage of the 2001 anthrax scare to understand how government health information is disseminated and how that information is utilized by the media.

The present study follows these lines of research by first determining how the mass media covered the 2003 SARS outbreak and then subjecting those findings to a normative analysis with the expectation that such analysis will provide suggestions for press coverage of any future global health crisis. In order to achieve these goals, we pose the following research question:

RQ1: What topics were prevalent in newspaper coverage of the SARS outbreak?

Additionally, this research should help us understand how newspaper coverage of a disease varies depending on both the level of infection in the community the newspaper serves and the geographic location of the newspaper. Thus, the following research questions are posed:

RQ2: Will newspapers produced in communities affected by SARS utilize different topics in covering the SARS outbreak than newspapers produced in communities not affected by SARS?

RQ3: Will Western Hemisphere newspapers utilize different topics in covering the SARS outbreak than Eastern Hemisphere newspapers?

This research also seeks to understand how newspapers utilize various sources when covering the SARS outbreak. Accordingly, we pose the following research question:

RQ4: What sources were used by newspapers when covering the SARS outbreak?

The issue of sources will also be analyzed according to geographic locale of the newspapers and whether the newspapers serve communities affected by the SARS outbreak. To provide this analysis, the following research questions are posed:

RQ5: Will newspapers produced in communities affected by SARS utilize different sources in covering the SARS outbreak than newspapers produced in communities not affected by SARS?

RQ6: Will Western Hemisphere newspapers utilize different sources in press coverage of the SARS outbreak than Eastern Hemisphere newspapers?

Episodic versus thematic framing

Media framing is the process by which the creators of media content decide to present or arrange a story in a particular way so as to suggest the "essence of an issue" (Gamson & Modigliani 1987, p. 143). Gitlin (1980) has argued that media framing is unavoidable because, at the institutional and individual journalist level, framing is necessary to interpret, organize, and understand large amounts of information. Media frames are ultimately about the selection and salience of story elements (Entman 1993), in that the process of framing involves both selecting what aspects of an issue or event is included in media content and the framing process also involves highlighting the specific parts of an issue that the journalist finds particularly relevant or important.

The way that an issue is framed has been repeatedly shown to exert an influence on the attitudes and belief of individuals (Levy 2002). An example of a framing effect is when individuals have different reactions to "logically equivalent" information that is presented with slight differences (Druckman 2004, p. 671). For example, individuals have been shown to explicitly prefer risk-averse outcomes compared to risk-seeking outcomes when the results of both options are actually the same (Tversky & Kahneman, 1981). That is, changing only the way an issue is framed can dramatically impact the way an individual understands and perceives the issue.

Working from the perspective that the way that an issue is framed is important, this project utilized Iyengar's (1991) model of media framing, in which media content is framed in one of two ways – either thematically and episodically – with *thematic frames* amounting to thorough, holistic coverage of issues at a societal level, and *episodic frames* centering on stories of the individual. The implications of the frame differences in Iyengar's model of media framing is an issue that is framed episodically is understood by the audience to be an issue rooted in the individual, that is, whatever is happening in the news story is related to the person to whom the event is occurring, and ties between the individual and any social causes or influences on that situation are left unexplored. A common example of an episodic frame is the case in which poverty is presented as happening to an individual so that the societal-level forces that may influence the individual's poverty are unexplored. Conversely, thematic stories, involve media content that constructs the issue at the social level, thereby exploring the ways that social policies and institutions come to bear on the issue being presented.

Iyengar found television coverage of many issues to be heavily episodic, resulting in news stories that put the blame for societal problems on the individual. While Iyengar's (1991) findings applied only to press coverage on television, Iyengar speculated that print media would utilize thematic frames more often than television. He also proposed that health issues – an issue not examined in his own research – would be the type of issue that would receive thematic coverage. Therefore, because print media is a communication form that is inclined to utilize thematic frames, and because it is likely that health issues are particularly conducive to the use of thematic frames, this research poses the following hypothesis:

> *H1:*   Newspaper coverage of the 2003 SARS outbreak will utilize thematic frames more often than episodic frames.

Method

In order to answer these research questions and test the hypothesis, a content analysis of newspaper texts on the SARS outbreak was conducted.

Data collection

The content analysis conducted here drew articles from four newspapers: *The New York Times, South China Morning Post* (SCMP), *Toronto Star,* and *New Strait Times. The New York Times* was chosen because it is the paper of record for the United States and is generally recognized as an elite paper. *The New York Times* also serves a city in the Western Hemisphere, a portion of the world that was largely unaffected directly by the SARS outbreak, though during the SARS outbreak it seemed reasonable to believe that SARS would eventually spread worldwide so that no location can be considered completely immune to the threat of SARS. The *South China Morning Post* was chosen because it is an English language paper in one of the SARS outbreak hot spots – Hong Kong. The *Toronto Star* was selected because it is the largest circulation paper serving the city with the most number of SARS cases in the Western Hemisphere (WHO 2004). The *New Strait Times* is an English language paper serving Malaysia, an Eastern Hemisphere nation that reported only five cases of SARS, while neighbors such as Singapore reported 238 cases of the virus and 33 fatalities (WHO 2004).

Thus, four papers have been selected that provide the data for analysis of how SARS is covered when the outbreak is local or not, and both of these conditions can be examined by newspapers originating in cities in both the Eastern and Western Hemispheres. Though the geographic distinction of hemisphere may appear somewhat crude as a boundary for the analysis conducted here, the reality of the SARS outbreak was that most of the direct threat from the disease occurred in and around Asia. Therefore delineating between Eastern and Western Hemisphere newspapers allows analysis to examine how press coverage of SARS differs between media sources that are located both close to and remote from the majority of the SARS cases.

Time period

Texts were culled from a time period beginning February 11, 2003, the first time the SARS virus was mentioned in any of the newspapers, and ending on July 31, 2003, the date that the WHO declared the outbreak over (WHO 2004). The Lexis-Nexis database was used to select all articles from the four newspapers that contained any of the following terms in any part of an article: *SARS, pneumonia, virus*, and *flu*. Only articles returned from this search determined to be addressing the SARS outbreak were retained for analysis. Furthermore, only texts appearing on the front page of a newspaper were selected from the articles returned. This approach has proved useful in examining news coverage of events in which the coverage was so prevalent or the time period selected was so large that an unmanageable number of articles were returned in an unmodified query (Menashe & Siegel 1998). Using the requirements for inclusion outlined here, a total of 288 articles were retained for analysis, a total sample that contained 181 articles from the *South China Morning Post*, 29 articles from *New Strait Times*, 49 articles from the *Toronto Star*, and 29 articles from *The New York Times*.

Variables used for coding

Five items were coded in this analysis: topics, sources, type of frame provided, the country featured in the article, and the date and newspaper of origin. Each of these will be briefly elaborated in this section.

Topics
Once all articles meeting these inclusion conditions were accumulated, one third of all the articles were randomly selected. Two coders analyzed this sample of articles in order to determine what topics were used in SARS coverage. Independently, each coder created a list of all topics encountered in the analysis of this sample. Once the lists were completed, the coders discussed each list, transferring topics that were agreed upon to a master code book and resolving any debate about the topics that were included on one topic list but not another. The end

product of this process was a codebook of SARS topics with robust definitions of each topic. This process of topic development has been used previously in determining frames used in media coverage of health issues by Menashe and Siegel (1998). From this list of topics, one primary topic was selected for every article in this study. Additionally, up to two secondary topics were selected for each article as was appropriate. In other words, every article necessarily has a primary topic, but the number of secondary topics varies from none to two depending on the construction of the article.

Sources
Up to four sources were recorded for each article. Sources are considered to be the entity to which any quote, paraphrase, or information is attributed.

Type of frame
Type of frame is derived from Iyengar's (1991) model of episodic and thematic frames. Episodic frames are event-oriented and use concrete, individual instances. Thematic frames place issues in a more public or societal focus. Thematic frames are usually more in-depth or interpretive. Following Iyengar's original method for investigating the prevalence of thematic and episodic frames, each article selected for study was coded exclusively as either thematic or episodic. Utilizing an entire article as the unit of analysis for investigating the prevalence of different types of frames was done with the acknowledgement that though "few news reports are exclusively episodic or thematic" for most media content "one frame or the other clearly predominates" (Iyengar 1991, p. 14).

Country of interest
Each article was coded for what country was being discussed in relation to SARS. Where an article focused on more than a single country, an International, non-country specific code was applied.

Date and paper of origin
Each article was also coded for the date on which the article was published and the newspaper in which the article appeared.

Results

Coder agreement

Twenty percent of all articles were randomly selected from the article population and coded by two independent coders. Using twenty percent of all articles for a reliability check follows social science research method guidelines (Wimmer & Dominick 1997). Reliability checks were run on each variable using Cohen's *kappa* (1968) a statistical test that accounts for chance agreement among coders. Coder agreement rates varied between .83 and .92, meeting the standards for high reliability (Popping 1988; Banerjee et al. 1999).

Topics

In order to answer the first three research questions, frequency distributions were run on topics by paper and for all papers combined (see Table 1). The first research question sought to clarify what types of topics were utilized in articles concerning the 2003 SARS outbreak. The most common topic found in this pool of SARS articles focused on statistical information describing the number of individuals infected with or dead because of SARS. Twenty-one percent of all articles coded included this topic. Numbers of dead and infected was an important and popular topic because statistics defined the status of the SARS outbreak. When the number of dead and infected was reported for worldwide levels, it presents the reader with a tangible construction of the nature of the global disease outbreak. When the number of dead or infected was presented for local levels, the statistics convey to the reader in communities intimately affected by SARS – such as Hong Kong or Toronto – whether the SARS outbreak is increasing, decreasing, or remains the same. In the communities that directly experienced SARS, the population monitored the daily number of dead and infected much like an anxious parent monitors a child's high-fever, constantly tracking the numbers and looking for any decrease that would indicate a break in the danger and a return to normalcy.

The second most frequent topic utilized in all the SARS articles focused on the isolation and quarantine that resulted from the SARS outbreak. SARS patients were isolated in hospitals, and in areas such as Toronto and Hong Kong, entire hospitals became quarantined, intended only for SARS patients. Additionally, in Hong Kong whole apartment buildings and hotels linked to the SARS outbreak were isolated and quarantined. The necessity of frequent isolation and quarantine in free societies indicates the seriousness of the SARS outbreak, and, as such, the topic was prevalent in the articles covering the outbreak.

Table 1. Topic distribution by newspaper

Topic	Newspaper									
	NYTimes		SCMP		Strait-Times		Toronto		Total	
	n	%	n	%	n	%	n	%	n	%
Dead/infected statistics	12	21.1	52	18.5	14	28.6	27	25.0	105	21.1
Isolation/quarantine	7	12.3	14	5.0	8	16.3	10	9.3	39	8.0
Healthcare workers sick/dead	2	3.5	27	9.6	1	2.0	7	6.5	37	7.4
How SARS spread	6	10.5	23	8.2	--	--	6	5.6	35	7.0
Policy on handling SARS was bad	–	–	26	9.3	1	2.0	6	5.6	33	6.6
SARS economic impact	4	7.0	18	6.4	–	–	8	7.4	30	6.0
Travel ban	5	8.8	10	3.6	–	–	12	11.1	27	5.4
SARS almost over	2	3.5	6	2.1	3	6.1	6	5.6	17	3.4
SARS impact on daily life	–	–	12	4.3	–	–	3	2.8	15	3.0
SARS impact on healthcare workers	1	1.8	7	2.5	1	2.0	5	4.6	14	2.8
Policy on handling SARS was good	3	5.3	3	1.1	5	10.2	2	1.9	13	2.6
SARS impact on air travel	–	–	9	3.2	2	4.1	–	–	11	2.2
Reports of mystery illness	–	–	8	2.8	3	6.1	–	–	11	2.2
How to prevent SARS in future	2	4.1	6	2.1	1	2.0	2	1.9	11	2.2
Treatment for SARS	–	–	8	2.8	–	–	2	1.9	10	2.0
SARS is new corona virus	2	3.5	3	1.1	–	–	3	2.8	8	1.6
Political impact of of SARS	–	–	3	1.1	–	–	5	4.6	8	1.6
Lack of disclosure about SARS	3	5.3	3	1.1	–	–	1	0.9	7	1.4
How to prevent spreading of SARS	1	1.8	2	0.7	2	4.1	1	0.9	6	1.2
SARS impact on sports	1	1.8	4	1.4	–	–	1	0.9	6	1.2
Benefits for SARS victims/families	–	–	4	1.4	2	4.1	–	–	6	1.2
People should not panic	1	1.8	4	1.4	1	2.0	–	–	6	1.2
SARS strikes kids	–	–	5	1.8	–	–	–	–	5	1.0
SARS origin in animals	2	3.5	2	0.7	–	–	1	0.9	5	1.0
SARS clean-up	–	–	4	1.4	–	–	–	–	4	0.8
SARS strikes healthy	–	–	3	1.1	–	–	–	–	3	0.6
Herbal remedies	1	1.8	2	0.7	–	–	–	–	3	0.6
SARS impact on immigration	–	–	–	–	1	2.0	–	–	1	0.2
Total	55		268		46		107		476	

NOTE. Topic distribution based on the results of two independent coders.

Other popular topics focused on issues such as the impact of SARS on health-care workers, narrative accounts of how SARS spread, various positions on the rightness or wrongness of public policies addressing SARS, the economic impact of SARS, and travel bans that were related to SARS.

The second research question was posed in order to assess whether topics would be used differently depending on how close the source newspaper was lo-cated to a SARS outbreak. Generally, all papers followed the same distribution frequencies of topics. Each newspaper, regardless of whether it was located in an area directly experiencing a SARS outbreak, used the topic of SARS dead and infection rates most often. However, moving past the most popular topic, some differences exist between topics used by papers removed from the SARS outbreak and papers located within a SARS hot spot. Additionally, the topics used by pa-pers local to the SARS outbreak are not perfectly homogeneous in frequency of topic use.

Articles concerning the illness and death experienced by healthcare workers from the SARS outbreak were much more prevalent in newspapers local to the SARS outbreak than the other papers included in this study. The *South China Morning Post* utilized this topic in 9.6% of all articles and the *Toronto Star* in-cluded this topic in 6.5% of all articles. These rates of use are much higher than in the two papers that were removed from the SARS outbreak (*New Strait-Times*, 2.0%; *New York Times*, 3.5%). The New York and Malaysia papers did not rely on this topic as much as the Hong Kong and Toronto papers because New York and Malaysia did not suffer the experience of large numbers of healthcare workers be-ing stricken by the SARS disease.

The *South China Morning Post* included the most articles (9.3%) with a topic criticizing public policies implemented to handle the SARS policy. For the *South China Morning Post*, this criticism was directed at both local leaders and those in mainland China where the SARS outbreak began. The popularity of this topic is a direct result of the seriousness of the outbreak in Hong Kong. Simply put, because SARS struck Hong Kong so severely, the Hong Kong and Chinese government were criticized for not doing something better or different to prevent the rampant spread of SARS. Alternatively, the *New Strait-Times* had the most articles using the topic that public officials did a good job handling the SARS outbreak (10.2%). The positive evaluation of public officials handling the SARS outbreak was natu-ral in Malaysia because even though the nation was located in close proximity to many areas where SARS was expansive (for example, neighbor Singapore) the nation largely avoided a SARS outbreak.

Whereas the *South China Morning Post* focused on bad SARS policies, the *Toronto Star* frequently utilized the topic of the economic impact of the SARS virus and the topic of a travel ban issued by the WHO resulting from Toronto being considered a hot spot of SARS. Both of these topics are related. As a result of the WHO advising the world to avoid traveling to Toronto, business and tourism decreased for the city, resulting in greater negative economic impact related to SARS. Hong Kong also experienced a WHO travel ban, but the *South China Morning Post* focused on this topic in only 3.6% of the articles included in this study, compared to 11.1% of all articles selected from the *Toronto Star*.

It is curious that the Toronto paper was so much more fixated on the economic impacts of the travel ban than was Hong Kong. A possible explanation for this disparity is that the Toronto paper did not perceive SARS to be as great a human threat as the Hong Kong paper did, and, as such, was more focused on the peripheral issues of economics. Hong Kong was generally more panicked than Toronto, and in Hong Kong the possibility seemed to exist that SARS could simply ravage the city's entire population – a possibility that makes economic issues seem less important than they would otherwise be.

The *Toronto Star* also utilized the "SARS almost over" topic more than twice as often as did the *South China Morning Post* (5.6% versus 2.1%). The reliance on this topic can be associated with Toronto's fixation on removing the WHO travel ban, thus lessening the economic impact of the SARS outbreak. In fact, shortly after the WHO removed the travel ban on Toronto, the city experienced a second mini-SARS outbreak (Donovan & Talaga 2003). The mini-SARS outbreak could be understood as the initial SARS outbreak simply winding itself out. However, the decision to remove the travel ban had already been made. A question worth examining is whether the WHO's decision to reinstate the travel status of Toronto was in any way the result of the "SARS almost over" message emerging from the Toronto media. Regardless, it is easy to see how focusing on issues such as travel bans and economic impacts can subvert the more important good of public health during a disease outbreak.

The third research question posed sought to understand if topics used in newspaper coverage of the 2003 SARS outbreak would differ according to hemispheres. In other words, would a newspaper produced in New York City (Western Hemisphere) utilize different topics than a newspaper produced in Hong Kong (Eastern Hemisphere)? This research found no differences between hemisphere-related coverage of the SARS outbreak. The absence of significant differences in topic use can easily be explained. First, the SARS outbreak was global (occurring in all hemispheres) and, as such, could not be relegated to simply being a geographically located disease. Secondly, massive public health threats, such as SARS, can be seen to threaten humanity in a very similar way regardless of cultural specifics, because the desire for health and avoidance of extinction can be understood to be universal values. Finally, though this research utilized newspapers from across the globe, each of the newspapers included in this study were based in, essentially, democratic locations. New York and Toronto certainly operate within democratic systems. Hong Kong, though it sits in the shadow of China, functions as a free society, and Malaysia functions with a semi-democratic political system and a market that continues to expand (Camroux 2001).

Sources

The fourth research question seeks to discover what sources were utilized in newspaper coverage of the SARS outbreak. In order to answer this question, frequency distributions were run on sources that were coded for each individual newspaper and overall (see Table 2). The findings indicate that the most popular source of information about SARS were government health officials, a group that made up 26% of all source attributions in the body of articles examined. Specifically,

Table 2. Source distribution by newspaper

Source	Newspaper									
	NYTimes		SCMP		Strait-Times		Toronto		Total	
	n	%	n	%	n	%	n	%	n	%
Government health official	16	17.8	92	25.5	23	45.1	32	23.9	163	25.6
Doctor	18	20.0	57	15.8	4	7.8	21	15.7	100	15.7
WHO	17	18.9	34	9.4	7	13.7	19	14.2	77	12.1
Government official (non-health affiliated)	10	11.1	52	14.4	4	7.8	9	6.7	75	11.8
Hospital administration	1	1.1	29	8.0	3	5.9	12	9.0	45	7.1
Citizen	5	5.6	20	5.5	1	2.0	5	3.7	31	4.9
Professor	3	3.3	22	6.1	1	2.0	1	0.7	27	4.2
Nurse	1	1.1	6	1.7	2	3.9	12	9.0	21	3.3
Business person	4	4.4	11	3.0	–	–	3	2.2	18	2.8
Scientist	4	4.4	6	1.7	–	–	6	4.5	16	2.5
CDC	6	6.7	3	0.8	–	–	4	3.0	13	2.0
SARS victim's friends/family	1	1.1	9	2.5	–	–	1	0.7	11	1.7
National leader	–	–	4	1.1	2	3.9	4	3.0	10	1.6
Economist/financial advisor	3	3.3	5	1.4	–	–	1	0.7	9	1.4
SARS victim	1	1.1	3	0.8	–	–	2	1.5	6	0.9
Flight attendant/pilot/airline rep.	–	–	4	1.1	1	2.0	–	–	5	0.8
Clergy	–	–	2	0.6	–	–	2	1.5	4	0.6
Doctors Without Borders	–	–	–	–	2	3.9	–	–	2	0.3
Athletic officials	–	–	2	0.6	–	–	–	–	2	0.3
Police	–	–	–	–	1	2.0	–	–	1	0.2
Total	90		361		51		134		636	

government health officials were local to the country being discussed; government health officials had ties to the health portion of government affairs and the ties were specifically mentioned in the article (e.g., Health Minister, Health Secretary). The government, then, was the entity most often responsible for disseminating the message on SARS. In fact, in addition to the 26% of all sources that were attributed to government health officials, another 12% of sources were attributed to generic government officials. This means that, in total, 38% of all sources were government officials.

Government officials are an obvious source of information about disease outbreaks because the government has, or should have, health data from hospitals, cities, and other institutions that, taken in aggregate, can provide an understanding of the true nature of an outbreak. Thus, government officials can inform the public of the nature of the health crisis and offer suggestions about what should or should not be done to protect individuals within the society. Using this reasoning, it seems natural for government sources to be the most frequently used sources concerning disease outbreaks.

However, this line of reasoning assumes that the government is offering unaltered disease information and making suggestions concerning public behavior based on a primary goal of protecting public health. Unfortunately, these are not always the conditions by which a government operates. During the SARS outbreak the Chinese government admitted underreporting SARS cases (Eckholm 2003), and the government of Toronto was accused of focusing on the city's travel ban instead of concentrating on the actual SARS outbreak (Cohn 2003). Thus, if media coverage of a disease relies heavily on government sources to define the disease outbreak and the government is distorting the true nature of the outbreak, social understanding of the disease will also be distorted.

During the SARS outbreak a global health agency, the World Health Organization (WHO), was the third most frequently cited source of SARS information for all newspapers included in this study. The WHO provided a sort of check on local government information about SARS. For example, the WHO was the organization that pressured China to disclose the true extent of that nation's SARS cases (Cohn 2003). Thus, in the 2003 SARS outbreak the WHO was able to limit some government distortions concerning the severity of SARS.

The final two research questions sought to discover if and how sources used by newspapers varied depending on whether a newspaper experienced a SARS outbreak locally or not, or if the newspaper was located in the Western or Eastern Hemisphere. The results of the research found that sources used by papers for either of these conditions did not vary dramatically. Overall, all papers used the same sources for stories on SARS. The most popular sources were government sources, medical sources (i.e., doctors, hospital administration, nurses), and the WHO.

Episodic versus thematic framing

The lone hypothesis posed in this research, that the 2003 SARS outbreak will be reported utilizing thematic frames more often than episodic frames, was supported. 76.4% of all stories selected for this research were coded as using thematic frames, compared to 23.6% of the stories that were coded as using episodic frames.

Three-fourths of all SARS articles covering the 2003 SARS outbreak were thematic because the outbreak was continually treated as occurring at the societal level. For example, as has been previously discussed, the most frequent topic in SARS coverage focused on the number of SARS victims. The number of SARS victims essentially tells the story of the SARS outbreak, particularly as the event is unfolding. The numbers illustrate whether the outbreak is expanding or decreasing and also provide a sense of how serious the outbreak is; the statistics of a disease are characteristics of the societal construction of the disease, and, as such, are inherently thematic frames. Much less frequently were SARS victims treated as individuals, which is an episodic frame.

Iyengar's (1991) original model of episodic versus thematic frames was developed to illustrate that societal problems were often being constructed in popular media at an individual level, and, as such, societal problems were not understood properly. Thus, for Iyengar in regard to political and social issues, the thematic frame is preferable to the episodic frame. We do not disagree with this contention; however, in regards to health issues or disease outbreaks, the episodic frame seems to be very useful in conveying the seriousness of the disease and creating empathy with victims. Episodic SARS articles in this study include texts with headlines such as "Nurse to abort baby after being infected with SARS," (Moy 2003) "Mother dies of SARS, baby survives" (Benitez 2003), and "Loss of both parents haunts SARS survivor" (Lee 2003). A cursory reading of only these few headlines, even in absence of the entire texts, illustrate SARS narratives that convey the impact and threat the SARS disease on the individual. This type of text is very different from the majority of the SARS texts, which discuss SARS statistics and the specifics of government imposed isolation or quarantines.

The episodic texts in the SARS coverage present a real disease that drastically affects the lives of individuals stricken by it. Conversely, the thematic SARS texts often hide the danger and severity of a disease behind numbers and guidelines. However, our point is not to say that thematic coverage of disease is unnecessary. Understanding how a disease is progressing and what must be done to prevent the disease is essential for a society to deal with the disease. Additionally, our point is not that the use of episodic frames in media coverage of health issues is perfect. Heavy use of episodic frames in coverage of some health issues may lead to a situation in which the victims of a disease become stigmatized, such as has been found to have occurred in media coverage of AIDS (Bardhan 2002; Clarke 1992). Our point is simply that there is also great power in the episodic frame for understanding the human experience of disease behind the statistics.

Conclusion

The 2003 SARS outbreak presents an opportunity to examine how the print media in several different locations reported a new disease outbreak that posed considerable risk to public health. This research sought to understand the media constructions of SARS by conducting a content analysis that focused on topics, sources, and types of frames utilized in press coverage of the SARS outbreak.

Our results indicate that the print media relied on thematic frames to present statistical information about SARS infections and deaths. Statistical information was used to define the nature of the outbreak, both in the disease's pattern of increasing or decreasing severity and in quantifying the literal threat posed by the outbreak. Print coverage of the SARS outbreak relied heavily on government sources for information. While this reliance seems natural, as governments should be invested in monitoring a disease and developing and implementing policy to handle the disease, it also has its drawbacks in that a government may manipulate disease data or base policies on goals other than public health, actions that, in turn, skew public understanding of a disease (see Gong & Dragga, this volume). During the SARS outbreak, the World Health Organization provided the valuable service of not only tracking SARS globally, but by also serving as a sort of monitor of national government health information.

Overall, newspaper coverage of the 2003 SARS outbreak focused on the number of disease cases and the reality of the measures taken to control the disease, such as quarantines and SARS victim isolation. Mostly absent from print coverage were sensational accounts of the disease or panicked constructions of the disease seeking to compel reader attention to the media source (but, see Hsu, this volume, for a contrasting example from Taiwan). This may be due to the fact that the level of panic associated with SARS, particularly in areas hard hit by the disease such as Hong Kong or Toronto, was already so high that the media transcended the urge to sensationalize. Or perhaps those creating newspaper articles about the SARS outbreak were, like many others, simply trying to remain calm and their texts illustrate that effort. Whatever the explanation, examination of press coverage during times of explicit panic deserves further examination. Events such as the dissemination of anthrax via the mail in the United States almost immediately following 9/11, or the terrorist attacks of 9/11 themselves would provide fertile opportunities to examine press constructions of events during panicked times.

Though this exploration of press coverage of the 2003 SARS outbreak produced several interesting findings, it also contains several limitations. First, this study dealt with only one type of media reporting of the SARS outbreak, that being newsprint. Further studies should take up the same questions posed here and apply them to all other forms of media, such as television, radio, and Internet (see Lee, this volume). Secondly, this research only dealt with SARS content from English language papers that served areas which were, at least somewhat, democratic. Further research should explore constructions of SARS in non-English speaking papers and from papers that serve non-democratic states.

Ultimately, the results of this research are important for the body of media coverage of health issues research because media coverage of the SARS outbreak was in many ways different than what has been found in research concerning AIDS, cancer, or heart disease (Bardhan 2002; Clarke 1992; McAllister & Kitron 2003). Whereas research on AIDS found that the disease was constructed as a health threat based upon membership in a specific "risk group" as opposed to specific risk behaviors (Bardhan 2002), media coverage of SARS was most often constructed as happening on a social level. SARS was usually depicted as a threat to all and the disease was depicted by the casualty numbers in order to convey to readers how the disease was progressing both locally and globally. Thus, during the SARS outbreak the media primarily focused on the movement of the disease across society, as opposed to the impact of the disease on the individual. The focus on society instead of the individual in regards to SARS likely has a great deal to do with the fact that the disease was, by all accounts, indiscriminate in whom it attacked and a threat to every single member of a society. Thus, individual behaviors or lifestyles were not part of the SARS equation because they had not been medically established as related to transmission of or susceptibility to the disease.

Also important are the results that illustrate a connection between the medical and the political. Government sources were the most frequently utilized in media coverage of SARS, and many of the themes in SARS coverage focused on government issues, such as praise or criticism of a government's actions to deal with SARS, SARS economic issues, and the level of government disclosure associated with the SARS outbreak. Thus, researchers looking at media coverage of health issues must always be aware of the possible influence of government messages on media constructions of health issues when attempting to understand how, and possibly why, health issues are formulated by the media in a certain way.

A final note about the results found here concerns the nature of SARS. The outbreak of SARS was sudden and devastating, and the eventual outcome of the episode was unpredictable. However, the outbreak finally dissipated, meaning that a cure or treatment was not found for the disease, yet it ended. This means that no one is currently suffering from SARS. So, unlike health issues such as cancer and AIDS, the issue of people dealing with SARS in the long term is not being explored in the media. Had SARS continued to exist in the global population in some sort of semi-controlled state, it might have eventually been constructed in a manner similar to other diseases. However, as SARS stands now it is in many ways an anomaly – a massive risk to human health that began, continued, and ended within a confined period of time. But, studying atypical health issues such as this is essential in expanding our understanding of the perspectives and diversity of media coverage of health issues.

References

Abraham, T. (2007). *Twenty-first century plague: The story of SARS* (paperback ed.). Hong Kong: Kong University Press.

Banerjee, M., Capozzoli, M., McSweeney, L, & Sihna, D. (1999). Beyond kappa: A review of interrater agreement measures. *Canadian Journal of Statistics, 27*, 3–23.

Bardhan, N. R. (2002). Accounts from the field: A public relations perspective on global AIDS/HIV. *Journal of Health Communication, 7*, 221–224.

Benitez, M. A. (2003, April 16). Mother dies of Sars, baby survives; Outbreak claims a record nine lives, including another three younger people. *South China Morning Post*, p. 1.

Bractic, E., & Greenberg, R. (1979). An analysis of U.S. newspaper coverage of cancer. In P. Hobbs (Ed.), *Public education about cancer: Recent research and current programmes* (pp. 53–65). Geneva: International Union Against Cancer.

Bradsher, K. (2003, March 31). A deadly virus on its mind, Hong Kong covers its face. *The New York Times*, p. A3.

Camroux, D. (2001). Malaysia: Winners and losers. *Asia-Europe Centre*. Retrieved July 1, 2004 from http://www.ceri-sciences-po.org/archive/octnovdec01/artdc.pdf.

Center for Disease Control (2003, September 29). Basic information about SARS. Retrieved December 5, 2003 from http://www.cdc.gov/ncidod/sars/factsheet.htm

Clarke, J. N. (1992). Cancer, heart disease, and AIDS: What do the media tell us about these diseases? *Health Communication, 4*, 105–120.

Cohen, J. (1968). Weighted kappa: Nominal scale agreement with provision for scale disagreement of partial credit. *Psychological Bulletin, 70*, 213–220.

Cohn, M. R. (2003, June 17). WHO rebukes Canada for SARS lobby. *Toronto Star*, p. A1.

Donovan, K., & Talaga, T. (2003, June 14). How SARS experts untangled the threads of the second outbreak. *Toronto Star*, p. 1.

Druckman, J. N. (2004). Political preference formation: Competition, deliberation, and the (ir)relevance of framing effects. *American Political Science Review, 98*, 671–686.

Eckholm, E. (2003, April 21). China admits underreporting its SARS cases. *The New York Times*, p. A1.

Entman, R.M. (1993). Framing: Toward clarification of a fractured paradigm. *Journal of Communication, 43*, 51–58.

Flay, B & R., & Burton, D. (1990). Effective mass communication strategies for health campaigns. In C. Atkin & L. Wallack (Eds.), *Mass communication and public media* (pp. 129–146). Newbury Park, CA: Sage.

Freimuth, V. S., Edgar, T., & Hammond, S. L. (1987). College Students' awareness and interpretation of the AIDS risks. *Science, Technology, & Human Values, 12,* 37–40.

Freimuth, V. S., Hammond, S. L., Edgar, T., & Monahan, J. L. (1990). Reaching those at risk: A content analytic study of AIDS PSAs. *Communication Research, 17,* 775–791.

Gamson, W. A., & Modigliani, A. (1987). The changing culture of affirmative action. In R. G. Braungzart & M. M. Braungart (Eds.), *Research in political sociology* (Vol. 3, pp. 137–177). Greenwich, CT: JAI.

Gitlin, T. (1980). *The whole world is watching.* Berkeley: University of California Press.

Iyengar, S. (1991). *Is anyone responsible?* Chicago: University of Chicago Press.

Lakoff, G., & Johnson, M. (2000). *Philosophy in the flesh.* New York: Basic Books.

Lee, E. (2003, May 1). Loss of both parents haunts Sars survivor; Yuen Kin-shing says the worst part of his tragic ordeal was not being able to say goodbye. *South China Morning Post,* p. 1.

Lefebvre, R. C., & Flora, J. A. (1988). Social marketing and public health intervention. *Health Education Quarterly, 38*(3), 24–25.

Levy, J. S. (2002). Daniel Kaneman. *PS: Political Science and Politics, 35,* 271–273.

McAllister, M. P., & Kitron, U. (2003). Differences in early print media coverage of AIDS and Lyme disease. In L. K. Fuller (Ed.), *Media-mediated AIDS* (pp. 43–62). Cresskill, NJ: Hampton Press.

Mebane, F., Temin, S., & Parvanta, C. F. (2003). Communicating anthrax in 2001: A comparison of CDC information and print media accounts. *Journal of Health Communication, 8,* 50–82.

Menashe, C. L., & Siegel, M. (1998). The power of a frame: An analysis of newspaper coverage of tobacco issues: United States, 1985–1996. *Journal of Health Communication, 3,* 307–325.

Moy, P. (2003, April 5). Nurse to abort baby after being infected with Sars; The powerful drug needed to save the life of the pregnant medic – who caught the disease from a patient – could cause foetal deformities. *South China Morning Post,* p. 1.

Popping, R. (1988). On agreement indices for nominal data. In W. E. Saris & I. N. Gallhofer (Eds.), *Sociometric research: Volume 1, data collection and scaling* (pp. 90–105). New York: St. Martin's.

Rogers, E. (2000). Introduction. *Journal of Health Communication, 5* (Supplement), 1–3.

Tversky, A., & Kahneman, D. (1981). The framing decisions and psychology of choice. *Science, 211,* 453–458.

Wellings, K. (1988). Perceptions of risk-media treatment of AIDS. In P. Aggleton & H. Homans (Eds.), *Health education and the media II* (pp. 83–105). Oxford: Pergamon.

Wimmer, R. D., & Dominick, J. R. (1994). *Mass media research: An introduction* (5th ed.). Belmont, CA: Wadsworth.

Winett, L. B., & Wallack, L. (1996). Advancing public health goals through the mass media. *Journal of Health Communication, 1,* 173–196.

World Health Organization (2004, April 21). Summary of probable SARS cases with onset of illness from 1 November 2002 to 31 July 2003. Retrieved July 2, 2004 from http://www.who.int/ /csr/sars/country/table2004_04_21/en/

Ying, L. W., & Lee, E. (2003, February 11). Panic grips Guangdong as mystery pneumonia-like virus kills 6. *South China Morning Post,* p. 1.

CHAPTER 12

Effects of rationality and story attributes on SARS perception

Shuhua Zhou, Chia-hsin Pan and Xin Zhong
University of Alabama / Chinese Culture University Taiwan /
Renmin University PRC

Social perception and the construction of social reality are intrinsically linked. This study tested the conjoint effects of participant rationality and two story attributes, severity and context, on perception of the SARS threat and on story evaluation. Participants' rationality was assessed by the Rational-Experiential Inventory. Stories of SARS were manipulated to be either severe or non-severe, and with or without context. Two experiments using identical manipulations and measurement instruments were conducted, one in the US and one in China. Among high rationality individuals, contextual information was effective in assuaging apprehension, but only in China where the perceived threat was serious. However, story attributes consistently affected story evaluation. Findings were discussed in terms of how rationality affected health information processing in response to changes in perceived risks and how story attributes contribute to the effectiveness of health communication. Implications for social construction of health risks were then offered.

Communicating the nature and consequences of health risks is one of the most problematic areas for media professionals, as well as being an understudied area for media researchers. However, the stakes riding on public understanding are high for those who create the risks, those who communicate the risks, and those who consume information about the risks. Unfortunately, as practiced today, risk communication is often very earnest, but also occasionally ad hoc (Morgan, Fischhoff, Bostrom, & Atman 2002). The outbreak of SARS was a case in point.

SARS was first reported from China in February 2003. The mysterious epidemic swiftly spread to more than 30 countries, killing nearly 800 people and infecting more than 8,000. The epidemic impacted Asian markets, brought a halt to its tourist business, and spread panic throughout the rest of the world. In mid-March 2003, the World Health Organization issued an emergency travel warning, identified the illness as SARS, and called for global cooperation to stop it. The epidemic finally faded in late June (Fleck 2003). The latest outbreak occurred in April 2004, at a laboratory in Beijing, China, which infected 9 people and killed one of them (Fleck 2004).

During the course of the epidemic, people had diverse perceptions of and reactions to the outbreak. Some panicked; many lived in tension, anxiety and fear. Yet others acted as if it were someone else's problem. Although many factors contributed to the assortment of perceptions, this chapter focuses on the personality of the perceiver and the role of the media.

Perceptions of SARS and the construction of the SARS reality, as with any health-related subject, are embedded in a complex cognitive tapestry in which differing cultures, experiences and values are at play. On the one hand, individual differences in the way people process information may play a key role in determining to what extent they will experience apprehension in response to a health risk such as SARS. Particularly germane to differences in information processing is the work on dual processing, or the extent a person relies on rational or experiential processing. Highly rational individuals may process SARS information differently than highly experiential individuals. On the other hand, when people are asked to estimate risks in the environment, most people usually have quite erroneous notions about them, often motivated by recent media coverage (Griffiths & Saunders 1997). The mass media play an important role in influencing people's perception, especially in times of high uncertainty, because an issue can be manipulated to sound more or less severe than it is. Reporters can also choose whether to provide contextual information on an issue or not. Research on basic perception and cognition has shown that biased media coverage and misleading personal experiences induce risks to be overestimated or underestimated (Slovic 1987), leading to skewed construction of such risks.

Literature review

Construction of SARS can be explained by looking at factors influencing the perception of SARS. The approach of this chapter is to look at the perceiver and the perceived. For the former, we focus on the perceiver's cognitive style and for the latter, the message attributes. At the center of cognitive style is the role of rationality in information processing. Its interaction with story attributes in affecting perception may offer an intricate picture of how SARS, or any other health risks, is constructed and consequentially perceived.

Rationality

When people face an epidemic such as SARS, how do they handle the dread, lack of control, high fatalities, and catastrophic potential associated with it? Cognitive and social psychologists have proposed a number of dual-process models for imagining the complexities of human information processing as happening along a continuum. Over the last three decades, the dual-process models have spawned a number of theories under its umbrella. Among them are the elaboration likelihood model (Petty & Cacioppo 1984), the heuristic-systematic model (Chaiken 1980), the continuum model (Fiske & Neuberg 1990; Petty & Cacioppo 1984) and the cognitive-experiential self-theory (Epstein 1994; Epstein & Pacini 1999).

All of these competing theories assume people use both rational and irrational processing when new information is encountered. But they focus on different targets. The elaboration likelihood model considers two routes to persuasion, central and peripheral. The heuristic-systematic model considers two basic modes, heuristic and analytical, by which perceivers may determine their attitudes and other social judgments. The continuum model tries to synthesize the two opposing views of processing, pitting elemental, algebraic approaches against holistic, configural approaches (Fiske, Lin, & Neuberg 1999). The cognitive-experiential self-theory (CEST) looks at the personality of the self and considers the rational and irrational styles by which an individual processes new information. The CEST has developed and tested sets of personality measures regarding the dual processes. It is therefore directly relevant to this investigation.

According to Epstein and Pacini (1999), people adapt to their environments by means of two information-processing systems: a preconscious experiential system and a primarily conscious rational system. The two systems operate in parallel and are interactive. The *rational* system operates through a person's understanding of logical rules of inference, a deliberative, analytical system that operates primarily in the medium of language and is relatively affect-free. In contrast, the *experiential* system encodes information in a concrete, holistic, primarily non-verbal form and operates according to heuristic principles. Despite the limitations of such operation, it has the advantage of being far more rapid and efficient than the rational system for coping with events in everyday life. The operation of the experiential system is assumed to be intimately associated with the experience of affect.

CEST psychologists have devised the Rational-Experiential Inventory (REI) in accordance with the tenets of the theory to index individuals' tendencies to rely on the two basic processing modes (Epstein & Pacini 1999). This inventory consists of four subscales. Two subscales index an individual's rational thinking ability and experiential processing. Two additional subscales index an individual's tendencies in and preferences for rational and irrational thinking. These sub-scales are combined to form two major subscales to index rationality and experientiality respectively.

Story attributes

Whereas an individual's cognitive style may affect perception of an issue, attributes of a news story may also impact how the story is perceived (Grabe, Zhou, Lang, & Bolls 2000). Journalists, of course, are not just passive conveyors of information about health risks. They decide, usually according to more or less well-established journalistic conventions, what to publish and when to publish it. They decide how long the story will be and where to put it. They interpret and comment on the policy debates and the decisions that flow from it. In reporting a developing risk, they explain the risk itself and comment on it (Cohl 1997; Crossen 1994; Hsu, this volume).

Reporting risks, especially at times of uncertainty, presents further pitfalls for journalists. Dueling opinions and conclusions from the scientific community and the sharp disagreement they precipitate make for sensational news stories (Crossen 1994). Because no definitive answers are available at times of unusual risks, journalists have greater rein in arranging, presenting and interpreting raw information (Dunwoody 1999).

Tankard (2001), for example, noted that the ways the media frame a story had subtle but powerful effects on the audience. He contended that, to a great extent, journalists dictated news content and defined an issue through the use of selection, emphasis, exclusion, and elaboration. Tversky and Kahneman (1981) found that presenting the same information about risks in different ways altered people's perspectives and actions. Excluding information from a message could have considerable effect on how people interpret the message. A group of health researchers found that, during the presentation of benefit information in the clinical setting, the way information was presented had significant effects on the decisions made (Edwards, Elwyn, Covey, Matthews, & Pill 2001). The largest effects were evident when relative risk information was presented. Their study also suggested that providing more information, more understandable to the patient, was associated with improved patient knowledge and a greater awareness of treatment effects.

Indeed, past research indicated that contextual information was directly related to perceivers' general picture of the issue at hand. Several experiments by Berger and colleagues found that people who were provided with background or base-rate data indicative of a risk manifested lower levels of apprehension and victimization risk than people not exposed to such data about threatening phenomena (Berger 1998, 2000, 2002; Berger, Johnson, & Lee 2003). Valenti and Wilkins (1995) concluded that journalists who produced longer pieces with context were likely to make audience treat the subject of the story as an issue rather than a news event.

On the other hand, the pursuit of sensationalism often resulted in making a risk seem more severe than it was. With the magnitude of an epidemic such as SARS, it was also easy to overstate the significance of any particular episode associated with the pandemic. From the perspective of story production, journalists often added dramatic forces to their stories in the way they arranged information to support a plot, narration, mood and perspective so as to attract and sustain attention (Berner 1988; Grabe, Zhou, & Barnett 2001; Grabe et al. 2000). As Rosenthal (1999) argued, the dramatic story attributes helped render a more powerful depiction of the issue at hand, allowing a portrayal with intensity and focus.

However, representation of undue severity does not come without a price. Perceivers may interpret the more severe report of a risk as more threatening than it is, and so draw unwarranted conclusions (Weiss & Singer 1988). For example, Pechmann (2001) tested seven types of antismoking messages. Those using a more draconian tone increased respondents' perceptions of the severity of the health risks, though they had no impact on intentions to smoke. High threat appraisal resulted from perceptions of high severity and/or vulnerability.

Method

Based on the research and theory reported above, this study manipulated two factors in the framing of a SARS story: severity and context. The first factor had two levels, severe and non-severe. In the severe condition, emphasis was placed upon the gravity and danger of the epidemic. In the non-severe condition, the story was more descriptive, without emphasizing the consequences of the epidemic. In the context manipulation, a *context* story put the SARS epidemic in perspective, comparing it to other deadly historical diseases whereas the *no-context* version omitted this information.

Two sets of dependent measures were used to evaluate the stories. The first set indexed participants' felt apprehension and emotion toward the stories. The second set was devised to assess participants' story perception in terms of journalistic performance, measuring whether journalists provided fair, newsworthy, and complete information for the consuming public.

Participants with different proclivities for engaging in rational thinking should perceive and respond to different manipulations of the SARS story differently. Given the nature of the rational system, high rationality people should be better able than their experientiality counterparts to recognize and integrate relevant information into judgments of their felt apprehension after exposure to a SARS story. That is, we expect high rationality participants to examine evidence and use logic in their response to a health risk and low rationality participants to use experiential and heuristic cues in forming their conclusions.

Theoretically, the more severely a story is framed, the more prominently affected the low rationality participants should be, and the more apprehension and emotion they should feel, because they are more likely to succumb to such manipulation without carefully analyzing the merit and validity of the information. On the other hand, participants with a proclivity for rationality should be better able than their counterparts with a proclivity for experientiality to discount the magnitude of a threat if contextual information is presented. When historical data is set up to contrast the relatively low severity of the epidemic, high rationality participants should exhibit greater reduction in felt apprehension than low rationality participants. Previous empirical evidence indicated that this was the case. Berger and his colleagues (Berger et al. 2003) conducted two experiments to examine the effects of participant rationality and base-rate information on apprehension about a threat. Results showed that high rationality individuals who first received context-expanding information about a relatively likely hazard (traffic deaths) manifested less apprehension in response to a subsequent news story about a less likely threat (anthrax death). Among low rationality individuals this relationship was reversed.

Accordingly, the following two hypotheses were proposed:

H1a: Participants of low rationality would perceive the SARS risk to be more severe than participants of high rationality in response to the severe version of the story.

H1b: Participants of low rationality, compared to those of high rationality, would perceive the SARS risk to be more severe in a story with context.

The traditional expectation of the press as the distributors of complete, fair and factual information to a public of inquisitive citizens seems at odds with casting journalism as an outlet for sensational stories. The focal point of discord is seated in departing views about objectivity: the traditional ideal of unbiased factual reporting devoid of unwarranted interpretation is not in congruence with the view of journalism as an attention snatch and drama machine (Grabe & Zhou 2003). Because the analytical style of high rationality participants is to carefully weigh the merit and justification of information and conclusion, they are expected to be more discerning in gauging the sensationalism tendencies of a particular story. Consequently, a story overstating the severity of an issue signals departure from the objective journalistic norm. A story without context, on the other hand, offers incomplete information for the more discriminating participants with a proclivity for rationality.

The following hypotheses are thus proposed:

H2a: Participants of high rationality will respond more negatively to the severe version of the story than participants of low rationality.

H2b: Participants of high rationality will respond more negatively to the no-context version of the story than participants of low rationality.

A story about a second possible outbreak of SARS was employed as the focal threat to test these hypotheses. Two experiments were conducted, the first in mid-August, 2003, in the United States and the second in mid-July, 2004, in Beijing, China. The second was timed to correspond to similar, relatively calm times in China when only a few cases of SARS were reported and a second outbreak was predicted to be possible. The second experiment enabled us to explore the possible effect of personal relevance because SARS affected many in China but few in the United States, even though it was billed as a global epidemic.

Experiment 1

Method

Stimuli construction
The stimuli were manipulated from a downloaded, two-page online news story from the Web site of the *Chicago Tribune*, which covered how health officials had cautioned about the possible resurgence of SARS and their plan to contain the disease after its first outbreak. The story also introduced the origin of the virus, explained how it had jumped from animals to humans, and reported the current infection and death tolls. Four versions of the same story were reproduced in Dreamweaver by keeping all the site features such as banners and links constant and by manipulating the subhead, picture used, lead, conclusion, and statistics to render the four conditions (2X2) for this experiment.

While everything else was being held equal, the high severity condition used a subhead: "New Outbreak Considered Highly Likely," whereas in the low severity condition, the word "highly" was omitted. In the severe condition, a picture was inserted which showed a masked nurse standing in front of a gloomy, deserted quarantined hospital room with a sign saying "No visitors allowed." In the non-severe version, a picture showed a woman reading a sign in front of a church saying: "Until the SARS outbreak is over, confessions will not be heard in the confessionals." In addition, throughout the text of the severe version, words such as "highly likely" and "urgency" are used whereas in the non-severe condition such words were replaced with "likely" and "conditions."

In the context condition, the story provided historical context of a number of catastrophic epidemics: the 1957 Asian flu, the 1968 Hong Kong flu (which claimed 1.5 million lives), the 1997 Avian flu, and the 1918 Spanish flu (with a death toll of 20 million) so as to compare the current death toll of 800 people. The no-context condition omitted such information.

Participants

In the first experiment a total of 237 student participants were recruited for extra credit, with 113 men and 124 women taking part. Most of them were undergraduate students enrolled in communication courses in a large US university in the southeast. The average age of participants is 22.6 (SD = 5.47).

Procedures

The study was conducted during participants' classes. After signing an informed consent form, they were randomly assigned to one of four experimental conditions with high/low severity and with/out context. Participants were then instructed to complete the first part of a two-part questionnaire. This part included 40 items of the 5-point REI rationality scales (Pacini & Epstein 1999) as well as some demographic questions. The REI scales measured participants' rational and experiential thinking styles. Non-significant and near zero correlations between these two scales have been interpreted as evidence for the orthogonality of the two information processing modes, which was true in this experiment (Pacini & Epstein 1999).

Participants then proceeded to read the SARS story in their assigned condition. Immediately after reading the news story, participants completed a series of 7-point scales measuring their fear and emotional responses, which included the following affective terms: overwhelmed, hopeful, angry, sympathetic, fearful, disgusted, uneasy, apprehensive, and sad. Participants then answered a series of questions, all on 7-point scales assessing the newsworthiness, informativeness, and objectivity of the news stories. To conclude the questionnaire, participants completed a battery of multiple-choice questions designed to test recognition memory of the news story, which is not reported in this chapter.

Index construction

The 7-point semantic differential scales of overwhelmed, fearful, disgusted, uneasy, apprehensive and sad were combined to form a relatively reliable ($\alpha = .85$, $M = 22.82$, $SD = 7.36$) apprehension index, which ranged from 6–42, with the higher scores indicative of higher apprehension in response to the SARS story.

The three items of hopeful, sympathetic and angry were eliminated from the index because they did not load well.

The 7-point semantic differential scales of newsworthy, informative, true, useful and new information were combined to form the other dependent index assessing the perceived newsworthiness of the story. The index was reliable (α = .83, M = 13.41, SD = 6.12) with scores ranging from 5–35. Higher scores indicated better newsworthiness evaluation of the story.

The 20, five-point rationality items of the REI formed a reliable rationality index (α = .85, M = 2.24, SD = .52), which ranged from 1.15–4.55, with higher scores indicative of higher proclivity for rational processing. The 20, five-point experientiality items were combined to form the experientiality index (α = .88, M = 2.47, SD = .58, which ranged from 1.00–3.95. This index was used to check its orthogonality with the rationality index. These two scales were not significantly correlated (r = .10). Therefore it was sufficient to use only the rationality index in the analyses.

Results

H1a predicted that participants of low rationality would perceive the SARS risk to be more severe than participants of high rationality in response to the severe version of the story. To test this hypothesis, A 2 X 2 ANOVA testing the interaction between rationality and severity was computed using a median split of rationality and the two conditions of severity as independent variables and the apprehension index as the dependent variable. No significant main effect and interaction were found. This hypothesis was therefore not supported.

H1b predicted that participants of low rationality, compared to those of high rationality, would perceive the SARS risk to be more severe in a story with context, because high rationality participants were better able to integrate contextual information to make severity judgments. A similar ANOVA to that of H1a was computed, substituting severity with context. Results also failed to support this hypothesis as no main effect and interaction were found.

H2a predicted that participants of high rationality would respond more negatively to the severe version of the story than participants of low rationality because of its perceived sensationalistic approach. The main effect for severity was significant, $F(1, 236) = 4.36, p < .05, \eta^2 = .02$. Participants perceived the non-severe version of the SARS story to be better than the severe version ($M = 14.24$, $SD = 6.43$ vs. $M = 12.58, SD = 5.70$). However, there was no significant main effect for rationality. Neither was there significant interaction between rationality and severity.

H2b predicted that participants of high rationality would respond more negatively to the no-context version of the story than participants of low rationality. The main effect for context was significant, F (1, 236) = 5.28, $p < .05$, η^2 = .01. Participants reported higher appreciation for the version with context than for the no-context version (M = 14.34, SD = 7.17 vs. M = 12.51, SD = 7.58). However, there was no significant main effect for rationality. Statistical tests also failed to provide support for any interaction between rationality and context.

Discussion

The first experiment was characterized by non-significant findings, except for the main effects of severity and context in participants' evaluation of the stories. In other words, apprehension was not affected by any of the manipulations. An examination of the rationality index showed a normal distribution, which meant that participants' rationality in this experiment showed a good range of variability. Theoretically, this variability should translate into different information processing patterns, such that higher levels of heuristic processing, rather than rational processing, leading to perception of greater risk (Trumbo 2002). But evidence of this experiment did not indicate that such was the case.

There were at least two possible explanations for these findings. First, the experiment was conducted in the US, with most of the participants being US residents. Because SARS affected mostly Asian countries, the cases of SARS in the US were rare even during the peak of the epidemic. It was possible that personal irrelevance might be a factor contributing to the null hypotheses. Moreover, time might be playing another part. The experiment was conducted in mid August, when the SARS crisis had almost completely calmed down. Even though the story was about a second likely outbreak of SARS, the fact that the worst was over might not concern most participants in this experiment.

To test these possibilities, a second experiment was subsequently conducted in China. We chose Beijing as the experimental site because the latest outbreak began there after two graduate students were infected while working at a laboratory with live SARS virus in March and April 2004. This outbreak infected nine people and killed one of them, with 862 people quarantined in Beijing and Anhui province. This small outbreak was contained by the end of May (Fleck 2004). For comparability, we waited until June to do the experiment to mirror the relative calm experienced in the US when the first experiment was conducted. A search of primetime television news coverage by ABC, NBC, CBS, and CNN through the online Vanderbilt University Television News Archive (http://tvnews. vanderbilt.edu) showed that during the period of SARS outbreak in 2003, US coverage peaked in April (N = 71) and May (N = 67) and decreased in June (N = 9) and July (N = 4). A search of Chinese television coverage of the SARS in 2004 by the only national network in China (http://www.cctv.com) showed that coverage peaked in April (N = 13) and faded in May (N = 5) and June (N = 1). Thus, it was within this general climate of reduced concern and coverage that the two experiments were conducted.

Experiment 2

Method

Stimuli construction
The stimuli were manipulated using the original English version of the SARS story, with outdated information on reported cases replaced by newer information on the infections that occurred in the Beijing lab as well as the fact that 862 people had been quarantined. Otherwise, the warning of a second outbreak, the explanation, and the conjecture concerning the possible origin of the virus were retained. Instead of the original *Chicago Tribune* website, the stories were embedded in the *People's Daily* website, downloaded with all the banners and links remaining intact. Again, the subhead, pictures used, conclusion and statistics were manipulated to create the severity and context conditions. For the severity conditions, the difference between the first and second experiment was the pictures used, because the first pictures were taken in a US setting. Instead, the severe version used a picture showing two masked Chinese nurses hurrying a patient to an emergency room against a backdrop with a huge sign saying "SARS"; in contrast, the non-severe version used a picture of people walking by an airport checkpoint which had a sign that said "Please check your temperature voluntarily." For the context manipulation, exactly the same manipulation was used. When all manipulations were completed, the four versions of the story were translated into Chinese to eliminate the problem of comprehending a second language for the Chinese participants.

Participants
A total of 200 students from a large Beijing university participated in the experiment, with 67 men and 133 women. Most of them were enrolled in journalism and mass communication courses. The average age of the participants was 22.9 (SD = 4.35).

Procedures

The questionnaire used in Experiment 1 was translated into Chinese. Back translation was conducted to ensure accurate rendition and equivalence between both linguistic versions (Triandis 1972). Otherwise the questionnaires used in Experiment 2 were identical to those employed in Experiment 1. Participants followed the same procedure as in Experiment 1.

Index construction

The same six semantic differential scales were summed to form an apprehension index ($\alpha = .86$, $M = 19.16$, $SD = 8.35$), which ranged from 6–37. Likewise, the same five bi-polar scales were combined to form the newsworthiness index ($\alpha = .82$, $M = 16.06$, $SD = 6.36$) with scores ranging from 5–35. The same 20 rationality items of the REI again formed a reliable rationality index ($\alpha = .86$, $M = 2.26$, $SD = .62$), which ranged from 1.00–4.35, with higher score indicative of higher proclivity for rational processing. The 20 experientiality items were combined to form the experientiality index ($\alpha = .83$, $M = 2.64$, $SD = .58$), which ranged from 1.10–4.65. This index was again used to check its orthogonality with the rationality index. These two scales were not significantly correlated ($r = .11$). Again, therefore, only the rationality index was used in the analyses.

Results

An identical 2 X 2 ANOVA testing the interaction between rationality and severity on apprehension was computed for H1a. The main effect for severity was significant, $F(1, 199) = 8.72$, $p < .05$, $\eta^2 = .04$. Participants reported higher apprehension in response to the severe version of the SARS story than to the non-severe version ($M = 20.84$, $SD = 7.69$ vs. $M = 17.39$, $SD = 8.28$). There was no significant main effect for rationality and no significant interaction between rationality and severity.

H1b predicted that participants of low rationality, compared to those of high rationality, would perceive the SARS risk to be more severe in a story with context. The same ANOVA testing rationality and context was performed. The main effect for context was significant, $F(1, 199) = 6.72$, $p < .01$, $\eta^2 = .03$. Participants reported higher apprehension in response to the no-context version of the SARS story than the version with context ($M = 20.55$, $SD = 7.69$ vs. $M = 17.39$, $SD = 7.52$). A significant interaction between context and rationality was also found, $F(1, 199) = 4.46$, $p < .05$, $\eta^2 = .02$. Follow-up t-tests were computed to decompose the significant interaction (Winer, Brown, & Michels 1991). These tests showed that among high rationality participants, individuals who were exposed to the

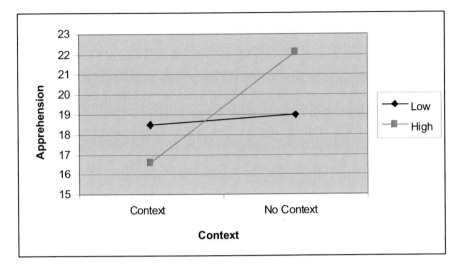

Figure 1. Rationality and context interaction on apprehension

context version of the SARS story reported significantly less apprehension than those who were exposed to the no-context version t (198) = 1.92, p < .05, one-tailed (M = 22.01, SD = 6.59 vs. M = 16.61, SD = 5.72, see Figure 1).

H2a predicted that participants of high rationality would respond more negatively to the severe version of the story than participants of low rationality because they were better able to discern the unwarranted claims. The main effect for rationality was significant, F (1, 199) = 6.10, p < .05, η^2 = .03. High rationality participants actually gave stories higher ratings than those with a proclivity for experiential processing (M = 17.21, SD = 6.34 vs. M = 15.00, SD = 6.57). There was no significant main effect for severity on story evaluation. Neither was there significant interaction between rationality and severity.

H2b predicted that participants of high rationality would be more critical of the no-context version of the story than participants of low rationality. The main effect for rationality was significant, F (1, 199) = 5.22, p < .05, η^2 = .03. Higher rationality participants were generally more appreciative of the stories than lower rationality participants (M = 17.12, SD = 6.27 vs. M = 15.12, SD = 5.78). There was also a main effect for context, F (1, 199) = 5.01, p < .05, η^2 = .03. Stories with context were better evaluated than those without context (M = 17.14, SD = 5.71 vs. M = 15.14, SD = 7.28). However, statistical tests revealed no significant interaction between rationality and context on story evaluation.

Discussion

Compared to the results of Experiment 1, which showed no main effects or interaction on participants' apprehension, the two manipulations of severity and context in this experiment both had main effects on apprehension. The severity version of the story and the no context version both generated more apprehension than their respective counterparts. In addition, the interaction between context and rationality painted an intriguing picture of how personality interacted with story attributes in the processing of risk information. Among participants with a proclivity for rational processing, story context played an important role in assuaging apprehension in response to the SARS risk.

In terms of story evaluation, it's interesting to note that high rationality participants reacted more positively to the SARS stories than their low rationality counterparts. Though we did not specifically hypothesize that high rationality participants would be more critical of the stories, it was theoretically implied in the interaction hypotheses. Results of this experiment, however, did not support this assumption. One possible explanation was that SARS was an acute epidemic; therefore, any serious story about its current status and a lucid explanation of the virus' origin were perceived by high rationality participants to be timely and necessary, whereas low rationality individuals evaluate the SARS stories as any other stories, without giving consideration to its social significance. If this explanation holds, it will complicate the role of rationality even further, because this argument effectively places rationality beyond the realm of stimuli by extending its role to the social setting. Instead of stating that rationality facilitates the logical processing of stimulus information, it also argues that rationality enables participants to assimilate other pertinent information, such as social significance.

Results on the context manipulation in the first experiment were replicated in the second experiment. Presentation of contextual information on historical epidemics as compared to SARS generated better story evaluation, confirming previous research on context and story attributes (Grabe et al. 2000; Valenti & Wilkins 1995). In spite of the main effects of context and rationality, however, data did not support the hypothesized interaction between them in predicting story evaluation. Context seemed to affect all participants, both high and low in rationality. Recall that context interacted with rationality in inducing apprehension. One potential explanation was that high rationality participants did indeed find contextual information useful, consequentially reporting more positive evaluation for the story with context, whereas low rationality participants might have taken a heuristic cue that the longer form of a story meant a more complete story (Valenti & Wilkins 1995), enhancing its perceived newsworthiness. In the case of apprehension, however, the heuristic cue of longer form did not bear directly on the notion. However, for the high rationality participants, the information contained in the context put them in perspective, which helped assuage apprehension.

Conclusions

Direct comparisons of the two experiments seem to indicate that apprehension was motivated primarily by personal relevance. In the US experiment, apprehension did not vary among all stories manipulations, arguably because SARS was perceived to be a remote threat. In the Beijing experiment, both attribute manipulations of severity and context modified the amount of expressed apprehension because SARS was too serious to be ignored at a place where most residents were affected one way or another by the epidemic. It also seems likely that personal relevance mediated the effect of rationality. The general increase in the perceived seriousness of the SARS threat from the US to China prompted different responses on the part of the low and high rationality participants. As Experiment 2 results suggest, high rationality individuals responded to stories with or without contexts differently, presumably because different information as offered by context generated more thorough processing due to the high personal health stakes involved, whereas among low rationality individuals, information was taken more at its holistic value.

Put another way, the reduction of the perceived seriousness of the SARS threat tended to erode the effect of rationality such that high rationality individuals tended to process information in more similar ways to their low rationality counterparts. Only in high relevance situations did rationality exert its influence. This notion conforms to the general tenets of the dual-processing theories that lean on the set of assumptions concerning limited capacity, least-effort processing, and attaining control. They all describe people as having a default strategy in which "truth" is achieved at the cost of systematic attempts to examine the data. Instead, heuristics, schemas, stereotypes, and expectancies are used to draw conclusions whenever possible, even among individuals with a proclivity for rational thinking.

In terms of story evaluation, results of these experiments suggest that attributes associated with a story continue to affect an individual's perception of its newsworthiness. The effect of the context manipulation was perhaps the most consistent. Stories with context were dependably rated better than those without. The significance of this finding is perhaps most pertinent to health related communication about topics such as SARS, because credible reporting often becomes the substantial basis of the public framing, perception and construction of health risks (Powell & Leiss 1997). Results of this study offer support to journalism scholars who advocate the provision of context (Gitlin 1980; Kovach & Rosenstiel 2001), arguing that a framework of interpretation is needed and reporting the facts alone is not enough (Tremayne 2004).

To what extent findings between the two experiments differ because of other confounding factors remains unknown. While we tried to keep everything as constant as possible, including the stimuli and measurement instruments used, the similarity of the media climate and comparable participants, we can not rule out the possibility that an experiment conducted in a different language, in a difficult culture, and with different pools of participants might introduce extraneous factors contributing to the dependent variables. Given the list of comparables, however, such a possibility seems unlikely.

At any rate, the proposition of immediacy and personal impact of health risk remains an intriguing one. On the one hand, when communicating a risk in the thick of a crisis, it seems that contextual information takes on increased cue value when the perceived seriousness of a risk is relatively high and personally relevant. However, it loses its cue value when the perceived risk is relatively low and personally irrelevant, at least among high rationality individuals, a finding corroborated by some previous studies (Berger et al. 2003). On the other hand, because it is possible that perception of risk manifests no effect once it's outside the course of the crisis and personal relevance, what can communicators do when they produce risk prevention messages, with the knowledge that most audience may be indifferent? These additional questions remain to be investigated.

One important task facing media researchers is to illuminate the processes that link media messages and social construction of reality. Unlike other chapters in this book which focus squarely on the social implications of SARS, this chapter attempts to explain how a health risk such as SARS is perceived and constructed by identifying relations between perception and reality. If all we have learned is that reality construction takes place in a health crisis, this does not take us very far. It leaves open a bewildering array of messages that are produced in many voices and many modes and that can be perceived and interpreted in many different ways. The assumption of this chapter is that those who bring something to the media messages they encounter, construct reality by negotiating it in complex ways that we are only beginning to understand.

This approach is useful for assessing relations among the beliefs held by one particular set of perceivers and the attributes of one particular set of messages. One of the major themes of social psychological theorizing and research has been that social reality is constructed by the people (Fiske & Neuberg 1990). Taking into account participants' idiosyncrasy in processing styles also assumes that media messages are open texts that can, and often are perceived and constructed differently. On the other hand, effects of story attributes have implications for the communication of health risks, be it SARS or the current Avian Flu. The way journalists arrange, present and interpret information may alter people's perception and construction of a health risk that affect policy debates and decisions that flow from them. Indeed, the stakes riding on social perception and construction of any health risk are high for everyone involved, including both journalists and information consumers.

References

Berger, C. R. (1998). Processing quantitative data about risk and threat in news reports. *Journal of Communication, 48,* 87–106.

Berger, C. R. (2000). Quantitative depictions of threatening phenomena in news reports: The scary world of frequency data. *Human Communication Research, 26*(1), 27–52.

Berger, C. R. (2002). Base-rate bingo: Ephemeral effects of population data on cognitive responses, apprehension, and perceived risk. *Communication Research, 29,* 99–124.

Berger, C. R., Johnson, J. T., & Lee, E.-J. (2003). Antidotes for anthrax anecdotes: The role of rationality and base-rate data in assuaging apprehension. *Communication Research, 30*(2), 198–223.

Berner, R. T. (1988). *Writing literary features.* Hillsdale, NJ: Lawrence Erlbaum Associates.

Chaiken, S. (1980). Heuristic versus systematic information processing and the use of source versus message cues in persuasion. *Journal of Personality and Social Psychology, 39,* 752–766.

Cohl, H. A. (1997). *Are we scaring ourselves to death? How pessimism, paranoia and a misguided media are leading us toward disaster.* New York: St. Martins.

Crossen, C. (1994). *Tainted truth: The manipulation of fact in America.* New York: Simon & Schuster.

Dunwoody, S. (1999). Scientists, journalists, and the meaning of uncertainty. In M. Friedman, S. Dunwoody, & C. L. Rogers (Eds.), *Communicating uncertainty: Media coverage of new and controversial science* (pp. 59–79). Mahwah, NJ: Lawrence Erlbaum Associates.

Edwards, A., Elwyn, G., Covey, J., Matthews, E., & Pill, R. (2001). Presenting risk information: A review of the effects of "framing" and other manipulations on patient outcomes. *Journal of Health Communication, 6,* 61–68.

Epstein, S. (1994). Integration of cognitive and the psychodynamic unconscious. *American Psychologist, 49,* 709–724.

Epstein, S., & Pacini, R. (1999). *Some basic issues regarding dual-process theories from the perspective of cognitive-experiential self-theory.* New York: Guilford.

Fiske, S. T., Lin, M., & Neuberg, S. L. (1999). The continuum model: Ten years later. In S. Chaiken & Y. Trope (Eds.), *Dual-process theories in social psychology.* New York: Guilford.

Fiske, S. T., & Neuberg, S. L. (Eds.). (1990). *A continuum of impression formation, from category-based to individuating processes: Influences of information and motivation on attention and interpretation.* New York: Academic Press.

Fleck, F. (2003). How SARS changed the world in less than six months. *Bulletin of the World Health Organization, 81*(8), 625–626.

Fleck, F. (2004). SARS outbreak over, but concerns for lab safety remain. *Bulletin of the World Health Organization, 82*(6), 470.

Gitlin, T. (1980). *The whole world is watching: Mass media in the making & unmaking of the new left*. Berkeley: University of California Press.

Grabe, M. E., & Zhou, S. (2003). News as Aristotelian drama: The case of *60 Minutes*. *Mass Communication & Society, 6*(3), 313–336.

Grabe, M. E., Zhou, S., & Barnett, B. (2001). Explicating sensationalism in television news: Content and the bells and whistles of form. *Journal of Broadcasting & Electronic Media, 45*(4), 635–655.

Grabe, M. E., Zhou, S., Lang, A., & Bolls, P. D. (2000). Packaging television news: The effects of tabloid on information processing and evaluative responses. *Journal of Broadcasting & Electronic Media, 44*(4), 581–598.

Griffiths, R., & Saunders, P. (1997). Reducing environmental risk. In R. Detels, J. McEwen, & G. Omenn (Eds.), *Oxford textbook of public health* (pp. 1601–1620). London: Oxford University Press.

Kovach, B., & Rosenstiel, T. (2001). *The elements of journalism: What newspeople should know and the public should expect*. New York: Crown Publishers.

Morgan, M. G., Fischhoff, B., Bostrom, A., & Atman, C. J. (2002). *Risk communication*. Cambridge: Cambridge University Press.

Pechmann, C. (2001). A comparison of health communication models: Risk learning versus stereotype priming. *Media Psychology, 3*, 189–210.

Petty, R. E., & Cacioppo, J. (1984). The effects of involvement on response to argument quantity and quality: Central and peripheral routes to persuasion. *Journal of Personality and Social Psychology, 46*, 69–81.

Powell, D., & Leiss, W. (1997). *Mad cows and mother's milk: The peril of poor risk communication*. Montreal & Kingston: McGill-Queen's University Press.

Rosenthal, A. (1999). *Why docudrama? Fact-fiction on film and TV*. Carbondale: Southern Illinois University Press.

Slovic, P. (1987). Perceptions of risk. *Science, 236*, 280–285.

Tankard, J. W. (2001). The empirical approach to the study of media framing. In S. D. Reese, O. H. J. Gandy, & A. E. Grant (Eds.), *Framing public life: Perspectives on media and our understanding of the social world* (pp. 95–106). Mahwah, NJ: Lawrence Erlbaum Associates.

Tremayne, M. (2004). The web of context: Applying network theory to the use of hyperlinks in journalism on the Web. *Journal & Mass Communication Quarterly, 81*(2), 237–253.

Triandis, H. (1972). *The analysis of subjective culture*. New York: Wiley-Interscience.

Trumbo, C. W. (2002). Information processing and risk perception: An adaptation of heuristic-systematic model. *Journal of Communication, 52*, 367–382.

Tversky, A., & Kahenman, D. (1981). The framing of decisions and the psychology of choice. *Science, 211*, 453–458.

Valenti, J., & Wilkins, L. (1995). An ethical risk communication protocol for science and mass communication. *Public Understanding of Science, 2*(1), 71–84.

Weiss, C. H., & Singer, E. (1988). *Reporting of social science in the national media*. New York: Russel Sage Foundation.

Winer, B. J., Brown, D., & Michels, K. (1991). *Statistical principles in experimental design*. New York: McGraw-Hill.

Index

In the series *Discourse Approaches to Politics, Society and Culture* the following titles have been published thus far or are scheduled for publication:

32 RAMSAY, Guy: Shaping Minds. A discourse analysis of Chinese-language community mental health literature. ix, 146 pp. + index. *Expected December 2008*

31 JOHNSTONE, Barbara and Christopher EISENHART (eds.): Rhetoric in Detail. Discourse analyses of rhetorical talk and text. 2008. viii, 330 pp.

30 POWERS, John H. and Xiaosui XIAO (eds.): The Social Construction of SARS. Studies of a health communication crisis. 2008. vi, 242 pp.

29 ACHUGAR, Mariana: What We Remember. The construction of memory in military discourse. 2008. x, 246 pp.

28 DOLÓN, Rosana and Júlia TODOLÍ (eds.): Analysing Identities in Discourse. 2008. xi, 204 pp.

27 VERDOOLAEGE, Annelies: Reconciliation Discourse. The case of the Truth and Reconciliation Commission. 2008. xiii, 238 pp.

26 MILLAR, Sharon and John WILSON (eds.): The Discourse of Europe. Talk and text in everyday life. 2007. viii, 200 pp.

25 AZUELOS-ATIAS, Sol: A Pragmatic Analysis of Legal Proofs of Criminal Intent. 2007. x, 180 pp.

24 HODGES, Adam and Chad NILEP (eds.): Discourse, War and Terrorism. 2007. x, 248 pp.

23 GOATLY, Andrew: Washing the Brain – Metaphor and Hidden Ideology. 2007. xvii, 431 pp.

22 LE, Elisabeth: The Spiral of 'Anti-Other Rhetoric'. Discourses of identity and the international media echo. 2006. xii, 280 pp.

21 MYHILL, John: Language, Religion and National Identity in Europe and the Middle East. A historical study. 2006. ix, 300 pp.

20 OMONIYI, Tope and Joshua A. FISHMAN (eds.): Explorations in the Sociology of Language and Religion. 2006. viii, 347 pp.

19 HAUSENDORF, Heiko and Alfons BORA (eds.): Analysing Citizenship Talk. Social positioning in political and legal decision-making processes. 2006. viii, 368 pp.

18 LASSEN, Inger, Jeanne STRUNCK and Torben VESTERGAARD (eds.): Mediating Ideology in Text and Image. Ten critical studies. 2006. xii, 254 pp.

17 SAUSSURE, Louis de and Peter SCHULZ (eds.): Manipulation and Ideologies in the Twentieth Century. Discourse, language, mind. 2005. xvi, 312 pp.

16 ERREYGERS, Guido and Geert JACOBS (eds.): Language, Communication and the Economy. 2005. viii, 239 pp.

15 BLACKLEDGE, Adrian: Discourse and Power in a Multilingual World. 2005. x, 252 pp.

14 DIJK, Teun A. van: Racism and Discourse in Spain and Latin America. 2005. xii, 198 pp.

13 WODAK, Ruth and Paul CHILTON (eds.): A New Agenda in (Critical) Discourse Analysis. Theory, methodology and interdisciplinarity. 2005. xviii, 320 pp.

12 GRILLO, Eric (ed.): Power Without Domination. Dialogism and the empowering property of communication. 2005. xviii, 247 pp.

11 MUNTIGL, Peter: Narrative Counselling. Social and linguistic processes of change. 2004. x, 347 pp.

10 BAYLEY, Paul (ed.): Cross-Cultural Perspectives on Parliamentary Discourse. 2004. vi, 385 pp.

9   RICHARDSON, John E.: (Mis)Representing Islam. The racism and rhetoric of British broadsheet newspapers. 2004. vi, 277 pp.

8   MARTIN, J.R. and Ruth WODAK (eds.): Re/reading the past. Critical and functional perspectives on time and value. 2003. vi, 277 pp.

7   ENSINK, Titus and Christoph SAUER (eds.): The Art of Commemoration. Fifty years after the Warsaw Uprising. 2003. xii, 246 pp.

6   DUNNE, Michele Durocher: Democracy in Contemporary Egyptian Political Discourse. 2003. xii, 179 pp.

5   THIESMEYER, Lynn (ed.): Discourse and Silencing. Representation and the language of displacement. 2003. x, 316 pp.

4   CHILTON, Paul and Christina SCHÄFFNER (eds.): Politics as Text and Talk. Analytic approaches to political discourse. 2002. x, 246 pp.

3   CHNG, Huang Hoon: Separate and Unequal. Judicial rhetoric and women's rights. 2002. viii, 157 pp.

2   LITOSSELITI, Lia and Jane SUNDERLAND (eds.): Gender Identity and Discourse Analysis. 2002. viii, 336 pp.

1   GELBER, Katharine: Speaking Back. The free speech versus hate speech debate. 2002. xiv, 177 pp.